2015

The Year Book of PLASTIC AND AESTHETIC SURGERY™

Editor-in-Chief

Stephen H. Miller, MD, MPH

Voluntary Clinical Professor of Surgery and Family and Preventive Medicine, University of California, San Diego

ELSEVIER
MOSBY

ELSEVIER
MOSBY

VP Global Medical Reference: Mary E. Gatsch
Editor: Joanne C. Husovski
Developmental Editor: Casey Jackson
Production Manager, Electronic Year Books: Donna M. Skelton
Electronic Article Manager: Mike Sheets
Illustrations and Permissions Coordinator: Dawn Vohsen

2015 EDITION

Composition by TNQ Books and Journals Pvt Ltd, India

Editorial Office:
Elsevier
1600 John F. Kennedy Blvd.
Suite 1800
Philadelphia, PA 19103-2899

International Standard Serial Number: 1535-1513
International Standard Book Number: 978-0-323-35552-0

Editorial Board

Table of Contents

Journals Represented

Journals represented in this YEAR BOOK are listed below.

Aesthetic Plastic Surgery
Aesthetic Surgery Journal
American Journal of Otolaryngology
American Journal of Rhinology & Allergy
Annals of Plastic Surgery
Annals of Thoracic Surgery
Archives of Disease in Childhood
British Journal of Oral & Maxillofacial Surgery
Burns
Childs Nervous System
Cleft Palate-Craniofacial Journal
Dermatologic Surgery
European Journal of Plastic Surgery
Injury
International Journal of Oral and Maxillofacial Surgery
International Journal of Radiation Oncology *Biology* Physics
Journal of Bone and Joint Surgery (American)
Journal of Burn Care and Research
Journal of Clinical Epidemiology
Journal of Cosmetic Dermatology
Journal of Drugs in Dermatology
Journal of Hand Surgery
Journal of Hand Surgery (American)
Journal of Oral and Maxillofacial Surgery
Journal of Pediatric Orthopedics
Journal of Plastic, Reconstructive & Aesthetic Surgery
Journal of Reconstructive Microsurgery
Journal of Surgical Oncology
Journal of the American Academy of Dermatology
Journal of the American Medical Association Facial Plastic Surgery
Journal of Vascular Surgery Venous and Lymphatic Disorders
Laryngoscope
Microsurgery
Plastic and Reconstructive Surgery
Revista Brasileira de Cirurgia Plástica
Sleep

STANDARD ABBREVIATIONS

The following terms are abbreviated in this edition: acquired immunodeficiency syndrome (AIDS), cardiopulmonary resuscitation (CPR), central nervous system (CNS), cerebrospinal fluid (CSF), computed tomography (CT), deoxyribonucleic acid (DNA), electrocardiography (ECG), health maintenance organization (HMO), human immunodeficiency virus (HIV), intensive care unit (ICU), intramuscular (IM), intravenous (IV), magnetic resonance (MR) imaging (MRI), ribonucleic acid (RNA), ultrasound (US), and ultraviolet (UV).

Note

The Year Book of Plastic and Aesthetic Surgery is a literature survey service providing abstracts of articles published in the professional literature. Every effort is made to assure the accuracy of the information presented in these pages. Neither the editors nor the publisher of the Year Book of Plastic and Aesthetic Surgery can be responsible for errors in the original materials. The editors' comments are their own opinions. Mention of specific products within this publication does not constitute endorsement.

To facilitate the use of the Year Book of Plastic and Aesthetic Surgery as a reference tool, all illustrations and tables included in this publication are now identified as they appear in the original article. This change is meant to help the reader recognize that any illustration or table appearing in the Year Book of Plastic and Aesthetic Surgery may be only one of many in the original article. For this reason, figure and table numbers will often appear to be out of sequence within the Year Book of Plastic and Aesthetic Surgery.

Introduction

Despite dire and imminent predictions of the likely demise of the hard-copy format of the Year Book of Plastic and Aesthetic Surgery, it has survived to live on for at least two years more: 2015 and 2016. Unquestionably, for most plastic surgeons, the computerized electronic format seems to be preferable. Yet, as in the publishing industry in general, there are quite a few people who prefer to have and use an actual hard-copy book. We will continue to accommodate this as long as we can justify the costs in providing both electronic and hard-copy versions of the Year Book.

We are delighted to welcome Thomas J. Sitzman, MD to our Associate Editorial Staff. Dr Sitzman is an Assistant Professor of Surgery and Pediatrics at the University of Cincinnati and is based at the Cincinnati Children's Hospital.

I would like to acknowledge the dedication and efforts of two of our Associate Editors, Karol Gutowski, MD and David Smith, MD. As in years past, both have done a superb job in their selections of material for this year's Year Book and for their cogent and wise comments and critiques. Much of their work and that of our new Associate Editor have been instrumental in increasing the numbers of articles presented in this year's Year Book.

I would like to thank Joanne Husovski, Senior Clinical Editor with Elsevier, and a new addition to the staff, Casey Jackson, Developmental Editor, who has done a superb job of organizing the materials with which I need to work in order to edit and organize the Year Book.

Stephen H. Miller, MD, MPH

1 Congenital

Auricular Deformities

Single-Stage Autologous Ear Reconstruction for Microtia

Kasrai L, Snyder-Warwick AK, Fisher DM (Univ of Toronto, Ontario, Canada; Washington Univ School of Medicine, St Louis, MO)
Plast Reconstr Surg 133:652-662, 2014

Background.—The authors have been using the Nagata technique since 2002. In this review of 100 consecutive ear reconstructions, the authors present technique modifications that have evolved over this period that have contributed to improved auricular contour and that now allow for auricular reconstruction in a single stage.

Methods.—This study is a retrospective review of a prospectively acquired database. The series is restricted to primary reconstructions performed for congenital microtia. Photographs of 10 consecutive patients are presented to demonstrate the results of the technique. Surgical complication rates are discussed.

Results.—One hundred ear reconstructions were performed in 96 patients. There were 75 primary cases of congenital microtia. Twenty-four ears underwent a two-stage reconstruction, and 51 ears were reconstructed with a Nagata stage I procedure or a single-stage reconstruction. There was a gradual shift in technique, with a trend to perform fewer Nagata stage II outsetting procedures and more single-stage reconstructions. In patients who underwent an ear reconstruction in two stages, the surgical complication rate was 22 percent. In the last 40 consecutive ear reconstructions since abandoning the two-stage approach, the surgical complication rate is now 15 percent.

Conclusions.—A modification of Nagata's technique of autologous ear reconstruction for microtia is described. Modifications of the three-dimensional framework address the contour of the inferior crus and control tragal projection and position. Inclusion of a projection block and recruitment of retroauricular skin allow for symmetric projection of the ear in a single stage.

Clinical Question/Level of Evidence.—Therapeutic, IV.

▶ Although a relatively uncommon procedure, auricular reconstruction captures the interest of almost all plastic surgeons. It appeals to our artistic sensibilities and combines our passions for aesthetics and reconstruction.

Costal cartilaginous frameworks are the standard for autologous reconstruction, yet no surgeon is truly content with the results of this procedure. This article provides an interesting and helpful perspective on how a surgical team learned from the masters, developed competence through clinical practice, and adapted their approach through critical analysis of their patient's results. Although surgeons actively performing auricular reconstruction may disagree with particulars of their technique, they will still be rewarded by a well-described surgical technique and a series of cases to which their own results can be compared.

T. Sitzman, MD

Current Management of Microtia: A National Survey

Im DD, Paskhover B, Staffenberg DA, et al (Univ of Southern California (USC) Med Ctr, Los Angeles, CA; Yale-New Haven Hosp, New Haven, CT; NYU Langone Med Ctr; et al)

Aesthetic Plast Surg 37:402-408, 2013

Background.—Microtia reconstruction remains one of the most challenging procedures encountered by the reconstructive surgeon. A national report on the current management of microtia has never been presented before. The purpose of this project was to survey members of the American Society of Plastic Surgeons (ASPS) to identify their preferences and practices and report their opinions regarding issues related to microtia reconstruction.

Methods.—An anonymous web-based survey consisting of 19 questions was distributed to the members of the ASPS. Questions focused on the management of microtia. The study design was descriptive, using categorical data analysis.

Results.—Thirty-eight percent of all respondents perform microtia reconstruction; 91 % learned the autogenous cartilage-based reconstruction technique, while only 16 % were exposed to alloplastic reconstruction. Seventy percent of all respondents learned autogenous cartilage-based ear reconstruction exclusively. Fifty percent of respondents who perform microtia reconstruction reported a steep learning curve. In the pediatric patient population, 49 % of microtia surgeons prefer performing the surgery when the patient is between 7 and 10 years of age, while 40 % of microtia surgeons prefer the patient to be 4–6 years of age. Fifty-nine percent of all respondents believe that in 15 years tissue engineering will represent the gold standard of microtia reconstruction.

Conclusion.—Staged microtia repair using autogenous cartilage remains the heavily favored method of microtia reconstruction among plastic surgeons. Moreover, there is a deficiency in training the newer surgical techniques, such as alloplastic and osseointegrated options. This study also highlights the continuing need to elucidate the optimal timing for microtia repair in the pediatric patient to mitigate the potential psychosocial morbidity well described in the literature.

Level of Evidence V.—This journal requires that authors assign a level of evidence to each article. For a full description of these Evidence-Based Medicine ratings, please refer to the Table of Contents or the online Instructions to Authors www.springer.com/00266.

▶ This report discusses current approaches to microtia repair. The authors queried American Society of Plastic Surgeons members using a Web-based survey. The response rate was 3% (n = 334). Only 100 respondents regularly performed microtia repair. This poor response rate raises concerns about whether the results are generalizable to all surgeons performing microtia repair.

The central finding of the report is that autologous reconstruction was more common than alloplastic techniques among respondents. Respondents were more likely to be trained in autologous approaches, and they tend to stay with that approach. The survey obtained other descriptive information about surgeon practices and beliefs related to microtia reconstruction. This information may be helpful in providing context to any one surgeon's approach.

On the whole, the article provides a snapshot of how a subset of plastic surgeons approaches microtia reconstruction.

T. Sitzman, MD

A long-term morphometric analysis of auricular position post-otoplasty

Graham ME, Bezuhly M, Hong P (Dalhousie Univ, Halifax, Nova Scotia, Canada)

J Plast Reconstr Aesthet Surg 66:1482-1486, 2013

Background and Aim.—Otoplasty is a common procedure to correct the shape and position of the external ear. Some surgeons have recommended overcorrection to ensure adequate long-term results but objective data are lacking in this regard. The aim of this study was to measure long-term outcomes of ear protrusion in children after otoplasty.

Methods.—All paediatric patients who underwent otoplasty from July 2009 to June 2011 were enrolled. Measurements of ear prominence at four distinct sites were taken intra-operatively and at 3 and 12 months postoperatively. Data were analysed with repeated measures analyses.

Results.—A total of 33 patients were included in the study, representing 63 ears. Mean age at surgery was 62.7 months; 20 patients were male and 13 were female. Participants underwent specific otoplasty techniques depending on the underlying anomaly (Mustardé suture placement, conchomastoid suture placement, conchal cartilage resection and/or lobular setback). Overall, there was no statistically significant postoperative change in any of the four measurements over time, indicating stability of the immediate postoperative result. No difference was also noted in any of the four measurements on the basis of patient variables or techniques used.

Conclusion.—Long-term auricular position, post-otoplasty, was found to be stable in our paediatric patient population, and therefore surgical overcorrection in the operating room is not deemed to be necessary.

▶ It is obviously important to know during the course of performing an otoplasty whether the ear needs to be overcorrected, that is, set even closer to the head in anticipation of drift postoperatively. Several authors have postulated that postoperative drift mandates overcorrection,[1,2] but these authors, in a careful, prospective, albeit small, and short-term study found that overcorrection is not necessary. It is a bit difficult to reconcile their results with those reported in the literature for several reasons, including the fact that the surgical techniques in other studies, as well as this one, varied among the patient population studied; the measurements in some of the other studies were from a single location as opposed to several in this study; and the short term for evaluation in this study. Obviously confirmation of this work needs to be performed and hopefully through a longer-term, multicenter, prospective trial. Additionally, postoperative evaluations should be performed by several independent evaluators and inter- and intraevaluator reliability assessed.

S. H. Miller, MD

References

1. Schlegel-Wagner C, Pabst G, Müller W, Linder T. Otoplasty using a modified anterior scoring technique: standardized measurements of long-term results. *Arch Facial Plast Surg.* 2010;12:143-148.
2. Adamson PA, McGraw BL, Tropper GJ. Otoplasty: critical review of clinical results. *Laryngoscope.* 1991;101:883-888.

Cleft Lip and Palate

Hospital care of children with a cleft in England

Fitzsimons KJ, Copley LP, Deacon SA, et al (Royal College of Surgeons of England, London, UK)

Arch Dis Child 98:970-974, 2013

Objective.—To analyse hospital admissions in the first 2 years of life among children with cleft lip and/or palate in England.

Design.—Analysis of national administrative data of hospital admissions.

Setting.—National Health Service hospitals.

Patients.—Patients born alive between 1997 and 2008 who underwent surgical cleft repair.

Outcome Measures.—Number of admissions, including the birth episode, and days spent in hospital were examined. Children were analysed according to cleft type and whether or not they had additional congenital anomalies.

Results.—10 892 children were included. In their first 2 years, children without additional anomalies (n = 8482) had on average 3.2 admissions and 13.2 days in hospital, which varied from 2.6 admissions and 9.2 days with cleft lip to 4.7 admissions and 19.7 days with bilateral cleft lip and palate (BCLP). Children with additional anomalies (n = 2410) had on average 6.7 admissions and 51.4 days in hospital, which varied from 6.4 admissions and 48.5 days with cleft palate to 8.8 admissions and 67.5 days with BCLP. The mean number and duration of cleft-related admissions was similar in children without (1.6 admissions and 6.4 days) and in those with additional anomalies (1.5 admissions and 8.5 days). 35.2% of children without additional anomalies had at least one emergency admission, whereas the corresponding figure was 67.3% with additional anomalies.

Conclusions.—The burden of hospital care in the first 2 years of life varied according to cleft type and presence of additional anomalies. However, cleft-specific hospital care did not differ between children with and without additional anomalies.

► This study quantifies the burden of caring for children with cleft lip and/or palate in the first 2 years of life. Using a claims database for all care delivered by National Health Service hospitals in England, the authors report the number of admission and number of hospital days. This all-citizen database overcomes existing limitations from previous studies addressing this question at the level of individual hospitals or for Medicaid patients.

The authors segment the population by cleft type and presence of additional congenital anomalies. The number of all-cause admissions for children with additional congenital anomalies was twice the number for children with isolated clefts. The duration of admission for cleft-related procedures was also more than double for children with additional congenital anomalies. This confirms the importance of syndromic status as a confounder when comparing burden of care and outcomes between patient populations.

In summary, the article provides valuable new information for anyone evaluating the burden of care experienced by children with cleft lip and/or palate.

T. Sitzman, MD

Reliability of Nasolabial Anthropometric Measures Using Three-Dimensional Stereophotogrammetry in Infants with Unrepaired Unilateral Cleft Lip

Tse R, Booth L, Keys K, et al (Seattle Children's Hosp, WA; Univ of Washington School of Medicine, Seattle; Univ of Washington School of Dentistry, Seattle)
Plast Reconstr Surg 133:530e-542e, 2014

Background.—Surgical and orthodontic treatment of unilateral cleft lip +/− palate can produce dramatic changes in nasolabial form; however, the lack of ideal methods with which to objectively document three-dimensional form limits the ability to assess treatment outcomes. The purpose of this study was to determine the reliability of three-dimensional stereophotogrammetry for anthropometric assessment of the unilateral cleft lip +/– palate deformity in infants before cleft lip repair.

Methods.—Preoperative three-dimensional images were acquired from 26 consecutive patients with unrepaired unilateral cleft lip +/– palate. Three raters performed indirect anthropometry on each image on two separate occasions, with at least 1 week between rating sessions. One rater performed direct measurements on participants before surgery while in the operating room. Twenty-six linear and angular measurements were considered, and intrarater, interrater, and intermethod reliability were assessed.

Results.—Regarding intrarater and interrater reliability, most measurements had Pearson coefficients greater than 0.75, mean differences less than 0.8 mm, and mean proportional differences less than 0.1. For measurements involving vermilion height, nostril remnants, or Cupid's bow width, Pearson coefficients ranged from 0.3 to 0.75, mean differences ranged from 0.4 to 0.9 mm, and mean proportional differences ranged from 0.1 to 0.3. Regarding intermethod reliability, correlation coefficients ranged from 0.4 to 0.75 for most measurements. The mean differences for nose and lip measurements were less than 1 mm and between 0.8 and 1.3 mm, respectively.

Conclusion.—Three-dimensional stereophotogrammetry provides a reliable method for many anthropometric measurements of nasolabial form in infants with unrepaired unilateral cleft lip +/– palate.

Clinical Question/Level of Evidence.—Diagnostic, II.

▶ Adding objective measurements to subjective assessment in cleft lip repair may substantially improve our ability to evaluate outcomes. Static measurements are difficult to obtain in this patient population, due in part to patient compliance with the examination and concerns about reliability. Stereophotogrammetry systems are hypothesized to overcome this hurdle by providing reliable measurements with short capture times. This study fills an important gap in knowledge by testing this hypothesis in infants with cleft lip and palate.

The author's findings are important for surgeons and scientific investigators. The intrarater and interrater reliability was very good to excellent, a reassuring finding for users of the system. The discrepancy between stereophotogrammetry and intraoperative measurements ranged by specific measure, and this has important implications for investigators looking to directly compare studies using these alternative methods of measurement. Overall, the study demonstrates stereophotogrammetry is a reliable method for measuring the cleft deformity. The results may lead to broader use of this technology for patient assessment.

T. Sitzman, MD

Influence of Objective Three-Dimensional Measures and Movement Images on Surgeon Treatment Planning for Lip Revision Surgery

Trotman C-A, Phillips C, Faraway JJ, et al (Univ of Maryland School of Dentistry, Baltimore, MD; Univ of North Carolina at Chapel Hill; Univ of Bath, England)

Cleft Palate Craniofac J 50:684-695, 2013

Objective.—To determine whether a systematic evaluation of facial soft tissues of patients with cleft lip and palate, using facial video images and objective three-dimensional measurements of movement, change surgeons' treatment plans for lip revision surgery.

Design.—Prospective longitudinal study.

Setting.—The University of North Carolina School of Dentistry.

Patients, Participants.—A group of patients with repaired cleft lip and palate (n = 21), a noncleft control group (n = 37), and surgeons experienced in cleft care.

Interventions.—Lip revision.

Main Outcome Measures.—(1) facial photographic images; (2) facial video images during animations; (3) objective three-dimensional measurements of upper lip movement based on z scores; and (4) objective dynamic and visual three-dimensional measurement of facial soft tissue movement.

Results.—With the use of the video images plus objective three-dimensional measures, the operating surgeon changed the problem list of the surgical treatment plan for 86% of the patients (95% confidence interval, 0.64 to 0.97) and the surgical goals for 71% of the patients (95% confidence interval, 0.48 to 0.89). The surgeon group varied in the percentage of patients for whom the problem list was modified, ranging from 24% (95% confidence interval, 8% to 47%) to 48% (95% confidence interval, 26% to 70%) of patients, and the percentage for whom the surgical goals were modified, ranging from 14% (94% confidence interval, 3% to 36%) to 48% (95% confidence interval, 26% to 70%) of patients.

Conclusions.—For all surgeons, the additional assessment components of the systematic valuation resulted in a change in clinical decision making for some patients.

▶ The evaluation of cleft lip repair remains heavily subjective. This is reflected in the poor agreement between surgeons on which children require cleft lip revision surgery. To reduce the subjective and variation in outcome assessment, the present study tests the hypotheses that adding (1) structure to the assessment and (2) objective information about lip movement can improve the evaluation. This is a valuable question for surgeons who are looking to critically evaluate their results and those of their peers.

The study's finding that both the operative surgeon and external raters changed their assessment after each intervention suggests that these interventions may be directly applicable to clinical practice. Larger clinical trials are needed to determine if this method of assessment improves patient assessment and, more important, patient outcomes. If substantiated in further trials, this method of standardized evaluation based on 2-dimensional and 3-dimensional imaging may become the standard for evaluating cleft lip repair.

T. Sitzman, MD

Prevalence, Cause, and Location of Palatal Fistula in Operated Complete Unilateral Cleft Lip and Palate: Retrospective Study

de Agostino Biella Passos V, de Carvalho Carrara CF, da Silva Dalben G, et al (Hosp for Rehabilitation of Craniofacial Anomalies, Bauru, São Paulo, Brazil)
Cleft Palate Craniofac J 51:158-164, 2014

Objective.—To evaluate the prevalence of fistulas after palate repair and analyze their location and association with possible causal factors.

Design.—Retrospective analysis of patient records and evaluation of preoperative initial photographs.

Setting.—Tertiary craniofacial center.

Participants.—Five hundred eighty-nine individuals with complete unilateral cleft lip and palate that underwent palate repair at the age of 12 to 36 months by the von Langenbeck technique, in a single stage, by the plastic surgery team of the hospital, from January 2003 to July 2007.

Interventions.—The cleft width was visually classified by a single examiner as narrow, regular, or wide. The following regions of the palate were considered for the location: anterior, medium, transition (between hard and soft palate), and soft palate.

Main Outcome Measures.—Descriptive statistics and analysis of association between the occurrence of fistula and the different parameters were evaluated.

Results.—Palatal fistulas were observed in 27% of the sample, with a greater proportion at the anterior region (37.11%). The chi-square statistical test revealed statistically significant association ($P \leq .05$) between the fistulas and initial cleft width ($P = .0003$), intraoperative problems ($P = .0037$), and postoperative problems ($P = .00002$).

Conclusions.—The prevalence of palatal fistula was similar to mean values reported in the literature. Analysis of causal factors showed a positive association between palatal fistulas with wide and regular initial cleft width and intraoperative and postoperative problems. The anterior region presented the greatest occurrence of fistulas.

▶ Palatal fistula is a serious complication of cleft palate repair. This study makes a significant contribution to the field by exploring the association of palatal fistulas with features of the perioperative experience. Among the factors associated with occurrence of fistula, 3 deserve consideration by every cleft surgeon. First, operative surgeon was associated with the occurrence of fistula. All surgeons in the study has > 10 years of experience and performed the same type of repair. Similar findings have appeared in cleft surgery and other surgical fields; so what is it that leads senior surgeons to achieve different results? The second and third factors answer this question. Among intraoperative problems that predicted fistula, mucosal tearing and suturing under tension stand out. Perhaps the differences between surgeons is caused by how careful they are to avoid tearing the mucosa, how they respond to a tear, and whether they accept closure under tension over increased mobilization of tissues (or delivery of additional tissue, such as buccal fat or gingivobuccal sulcus mucosal flaps). Although the answers to these questions cannot be provided in this retrospective study, they should be considered by all surgeons performing palate repair.

T. Sitzman, MD

Prevalence, Cause, and Location of Palatal Fistula in Operated Complete Unilateral Cleft Lip and Palate: Retrospective Study

de Agostino Biella Passos V, de Carvalho Carrara CF, da Silva Dalben G, et al (Hosp for Rehabilitation of Craniofacial Anomalies, Bauru, São Paulo, Brazil)

Cleft Palate Craniofac J 51:158-164, 2014

Objective.—To evaluate the prevalence of fistulas after palate repair and analyze their location and association with possible causal factors.

Design.—Retrospective analysis of patient records and evaluation of preoperative initial photographs.

Setting.—Tertiary craniofacial center.

Participants.—Five hundred eighty-nine individuals with complete unilateral cleft lip and palate that underwent palate repair at the age of 12 to 36 months by the von Langenbeck technique, in a single stage, by the plastic surgery team of the hospital, from January 2003 to July 2007.

Interventions.—The cleft width was visually classified by a single examiner as narrow, regular, or wide. The following regions of the palate were considered for the location: anterior, medium, transition (between hard and soft palate), and soft palate.

Main Outcome Measures.—Descriptive statistics and analysis of association between the occurrence of fistula and the different parameters were evaluated.

Results.—Palatal fistulas were observed in 27% of the sample, with a greater proportion at the anterior region (37.11%). The chi-square statistical test revealed statistically significant association ($P \leq .05$) between the fistulas and initial cleft width ($P = .0003$), intraoperative problems ($P = .0037$), and postoperative problems ($P = .00002$).

Conclusions.—The prevalence of palatal fistula was similar to mean values reported in the literature. Analysis of causal factors showed a positive association between palatal fistulas with wide and regular initial cleft width and intraoperative and postoperative problems. The anterior region presented the greatest occurrence of fistulas.

► Oronasal fistulas are a well-known complication of cleft palate repair. Rates of fistula vary more than 10-fold among earlier reports. The ability to identify sources of this variation have been limited because of inconsistent reporting methods, differences in patient characteristics between cohorts, and small sample sizes. The present study uses a retrospective chart review at a busy South American cleft center to provide new insights and confirm previous findings about the predictors of palatal fistula. Although the retrospective design and lack of a multivariate regression limits the applicability to prospective interventions, the results are important to consider.

The article has several notable findings that point the way to lowering fistula rates after palate repair. First, when performing a von Langenbeck palatoplasty most fistulas occur in or adjacent to the hard palate. Second, mucosal tears and suturing under tension are associated with palatal fistula, and these intraoperative issues should be avoided. Finally, there is substantial evidence that fistula rate is surgeon-dependent. Using this information, surgeons can evaluate their own results and consider what interventions could help them improve.

T. Sitzman, MD

Autologous fat grafting for the treatment of velopharyngeal insufficiency: State of the art

Bishop A, Hong P, Bezuhly M (Dalhousie Univ, Halifax, Nova Scotia, Canada)
J Plast Reconstr Aesthet Surg 67:1-8, 2014

Background.—Autologous fat grafting to the velopharynx has been described for treatment of velopharyngeal insufficiency for over a decade. The aim of this review was to evaluate outcomes of autologous fat grafting for velopharyngeal insufficiency.

Methods.—A computerized search was performed across multiple databases. Studies involving patients undergoing autologous fat grafting for velopharyngeal insufficiency treatment that reported at least one pre- and post-intervention outcome measure were included.

Results.—A systematic search revealed eleven studies that satisfied inclusion criteria. All were case series or noncomparative observational studies. Three reported on isolated posterior pharyngeal wall augmentation, while eight involved augmentation of the pharyngeal arches, velum and/or posterior pharyngeal wall. In general, selected patients had plateaued with regards to speech therapy and had small-to-moderate velopharyngeal closure defects. Although most patients had a cleft palate diagnosis, the proportion that had previous velopharyngoplasty, or other related diagnoses was highly variable. In all but one report outcome measures included perceptual speech assessment. Objective measures such as nasalance and fat graft take were inconsistently reported. Overall, results of fat grafting for velopharyngeal insufficiency were variable and depended on assessment modality. One case of obstructive sleep apnea was reported.

Conclusions.—Despite potential benefits of autologous fat grafting for velopharyngeal insufficiency, questions remain as to patient selection, safety, and optimal graft volume and injection sites. This review underscores the need for standardized assessment methods and prospective comparative studies or randomized controlled trials to compare fat grafting with established velopharyngoplasty techniques to better define indications for its use.

▶ This systematic review of autologous fat grafting for treatment of velopharyngeal insufficiency (VPI) provides important information on the efficacy and safety of this experimental procedure. Although numerous variations on posterior wall augmentation for VPI have been reported in the past 50 years, none has been widely adopted. Autologous fat grafting is the perhaps the latest variation on this theme, and this review provides a useful update on what is known about the procedure's efficacy. The included reports unfortunately provide few data about safety. Fortunately, the authors provide valuable references for case reports of known complications with the procedure, including blindness and stroke. This is an essential read for any surgeon considering autologous fat grafting for management of VPI.

T. Sitzman, MD

Impact of Sleep and Breathing in Infancy on Outcomes at Three Years of Age for Children with Cleft Lip and/or Palate

Smith CB, Walker K, Badawi N, et al (The Children's Hosp at Westmead, New South Wales, Australia; Univ of Sydney, New South Wales, Australia)
Sleep 37:919-925, 2014

Study Objectives.—To evaluate the relationship between sleep disordered breathing (SDB) in early infancy and outcomes at 3 years of age in children with cleft lip and/or palate (CL/P).

Design.—Observational follow-up study.

Setting.—Multidisciplinary CL/P clinic, tertiary centre.

Participants.—Children with CL/P who participated in a study of sleep and breathing in infancy.

Measurements and Results.—The families of 52 children were approached for this follow-up study. The children underwent neurocognitive (Bayley Scales of Infant and Toddler Development, Third Edition; BSID-III), quality of life (Infant/Toddler Quality of Life Questionnaire; ITQOL), and growth assessments at 3 years. The families of 33 children (66%) completed follow-up at 36.7 ± 1.4 months. The apnea-hypopnea index (AHI) in infancy was 23.9 ± 18.0 events/h. Mean group BSID-III scores fell within the standardized normal range (10 ± 3) for all domains; however, language scores were lower than control children. Quality of life scores and growth parameter z-scores were similar to published control data. PSG variables in infancy showed significant relationships with outcomes at 3 years of age; lower percentage of AS/REM sleep was associated with lower cognition score; more obstructive events were associated with lower global behavior ITQOL score; and higher number of respiratory events in infancy was associated with lower weight z-score.

Conclusion.—Neurocognition, quality of life, and growth measures from children with CL/P fall within a normal range; however, scores in the language domain are lower than controls. Sleep and respiratory elements of SDB in infancy appear to modify these outcomes at 3 years of age.

▶ Sleep-disordered breathing (SDB) is an increasingly recognized medical condition in our society. Children with cleft lip and/or palate (CL/P) may be at increased risk for SDB due to hypoplasia of the facial skeleton or mandibular retrognathia. This research team previously demonstrated that 40% of infants with CL/P had evidence of obstructive apnea during sleep. This raises the important question of whether the presence of SDB in infancy affects neurocognitive, quality of life, and growth outcomes later in life.

This is the first study to report long-term outcomes of SDB in infancy for children with CL/P. Most of the participants diagnosed with SDB in infancy did receive treatment, so rather than addressing the impact of SDB alone, the study compared the effect of SDB treated by pediatric sleep physicians to outcomes for children with neither SDB nor CL/P. This is an important distinction but does not diminish the importance of the study.

Overall, the investigators found that children with CL/P and SDB achieve "normal neurocognitive function, quality of life, and growth at 3 years of age." This is a reassuring finding for parents, who will take heart in knowing that their child's sleep apnea can be successfully treated. It also leaves open a door for future studies to determine exactly which children benefit from treatment for SDB.

T. Sitzman, MD

Cranio-maxillo-facial

3D stereophotogrammetric analysis of operative effects after broad median craniectomy in premature sagittal craniosynostosis

Linz C, Meyer-Marcotty P, Böhm H, et al (Univ Hosp of Würzburg, Germany; et al)

Childs Nerv Syst 30:313-318, 2014

Introduction.—There is ongoing discussion on the diagnostic methods, the need of surgical treatment, and the surgical strategies for premature craniosynostosis.

Materials and Methods.—This study examined the operative procedure of a standardized broad median craniectomy, active tilting of the forehead, and bitemporal greenstick fracturing in children with premature sagittal craniosynostosis. To objectively analyze the direct surgical results, we used a 3D stereophotogrammetry scanner, as previously described.

Results.—A 3D analysis showed a significant increase in the width, cranial index (CI), head and coronal circumferences, intracranial volume, and cranial base width after surgery. Head length was the only parameter that demonstrated a significant decrease postoperatively. Asymmetry and the 30° diagonal difference showed no significant changes.

Conclusion.—3D stereophotogrammetry is a reliable and valuable tool with no side effects. It demonstrated that the extended surgical procedure achieves good postoperative results with a reduced length and increased width and, therefore, an improved CI. Additionally, the total intracranial volume was significantly increased after surgery.

▶ This article is notable for it use of 3-dimensional (3D) stereophotogrammetry to evaluate changes in head shape after correction of sagittal craniosynostosis. As 3D imaging becomes more widely available, evaluation of surgical outcomes will be an important application. In the present study, the investigators used ultrasound and skull x-ray to confirm their diagnosis and 3D stereophotogrammetry to evaluate outcomes. They did not obtain computed tomography scan pre- or postoperatively. This article is worth reading for surgeons who conduct craniofacial surgery and are interested applying 3D imaging to evaluate their outcomes.

T. Sitzman, MD

Vascular Malformations

Atenolol versus propranolol for the treatment of infantile hemangiomas: A randomized controlled study

Abarzúa-Araya Á, Navarrete-Dechent CP, Heusser F, et al (Pontificia Universidad Católica de Chile, Santiago)

J Am Acad Dermatol 70:1045-1049, 2014

Background.—Infantile hemangiomas have a dramatic response to propranolol, a nonselective beta-blocker. However, this treatment is not risk-free and many patients are excluded because of respiratory comorbidities. Atenolol is a cardioselective beta-blocker that may have fewer adverse events.

Objective.—We sought to evaluate the effectiveness of atenolol against propranolol in a noninferiority trial.

Methods.—In all, 23 patients met the inclusion criteria and were randomized to receive either atenolol or propranolol. Thirteen patients were treated with atenolol and 10 with propranolol. Follow-up was made at baseline, 2 weeks, 4 weeks, and then monthly for 6 months.

Results.—Patients treated with atenolol had a complete response of 53.8% and 60% with propranolol, respectively. These results were nonsignificant ($P = .68$). Relevant adverse events were not reported.

Limitations.—The reduced number of patients could have influenced our results.

Conclusion.—Atenolol appears to be as effective as propranolol. We did not find significant differences between these results or any adverse events.

▶ The evidence for treatment of infantile hemangiomas with propranolol continues to grow. Results of phase 2 clinical trials show equivalence to steroid treatment, and many providers have already switched to propranolol as first-line therapy. Despite the promising clinical results, the mechanism of action for propanol remains incompletely understood.

It remains unknown whether the efficacy of propranolol is specific to this agent or applies to other beta-blockers. Two previous case reports suggest atenolol may also produce regression of infantile hemangiomas. The present study contributes to the field by providing a pilot randomized controlled trial of atenolol to propranolol therapy.

The results of this study suggest that atenolol is a viable alternative to propranolol. If confirmed in further studies, this could simplify dosing regiments and theoretically reduce side effects from beta-blocker therapy.

Interested readers should also see the recent cohort study by de Graaf et al[1] addressing this question. Although not a randomized or blinded study, the report by de Graaf includes a larger cohort of patients.

T. Sitzman, MD

Reference

1. de Graaf M, Raphael MF, Breugem CC, et al. Treatment of infantile haemangiomas with atenolol: comparison with a historical propranolol group. *J Plast Reconstr Aesthet Surg*. 2013;66:1732-1740.

2 Neoplastic, Inflammatory and Degenerative Conditions

Facial Nerve Paralysis

Rapid and Accurate Identification of Cut Ends of Facial Nerves Using a Nerve Monitoring System During Surgical Exploration and Anastomosis

Dai J, Shen SG, Zhang S, et al (Shanghai Jiao Tong Univ School of Medicine, China)

J Oral Maxillofac Surg 71:1809.e1-1809.e5, 2013

Purpose.—Surgical exploration and end-to-end neurorrhaphy is the preferred management for traumatic facial nerve injury. Traditionally, finding the cut ends of facial nerves depends mainly on a surgeon's experience. In this study, a nerve monitoring system to help the surgeon quickly and accurately identify, confirm, and locate the cut ends of facial nerve branches was investigated.

Patients and Methods.—Six patients with traumatic facial nerve injury were selected, and the nerve monitoring system was applied during the surgical process of facial nerve exploration and anastomosis. Operation time and surgical outcome were used to evaluate the effect of this method.

Results.—The surgical procedures required 6 to 15 minutes (mean, 10 minutes) for detecting and dissecting each cut end of a facial nerve branch. All cut ends of injured facial nerve branches were found during surgery in all 6 patients, and no intraoperative complications were encountered. The postoperative function of the facial nerve, evaluated by clinical examination and diagnostic electroneurography, was satisfactory and symmetrical in all 6 patients at 3 months.

Conclusion.—Using a nerve monitoring system could effectively help surgeons achieve rapid and accurate identification of the cut ends of facial

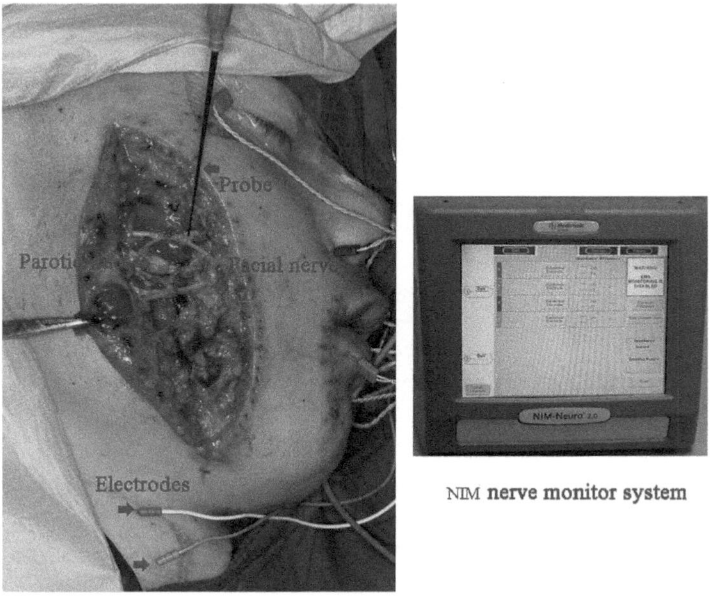

FIGURE 3.—Intraoperative photograph of case 1 displaying the probe of the NIM nerve monitoring system to detect injured facial nerve branches during surgery. (Reprinted from Dai J, Shen SG, Zhang S, et al. Rapid and accurate identification of cut ends of facial nerves using a nerve monitoring system during surgical exploration and anastomosis. *J Oral Maxillofac Surg*. 2013;71:1809.e1-1809.e5, Copyright 2013, with permission from American Association of Oral and Maxillofacial Surgeons.)

nerves during surgical facial nerve exploration for traumatic facial nerve injury (Fig 3).

▶ This study out of China reports very interesting technology. The authors describe the use of a commercially available nerve monitoring system, NIM-Neuro 2.0, created by Medtronic Corporation in Minneapolis, MN. The device was used to identify the cut ends of facial nerves within a short period, averaging 10 minutes, and was successful in all 6 patients in whom it was used. Certainly, those of us who have spent much time searching for the cut ends of the facial nerve would appreciate having such a device available. It would obviously be useful in many other situations in which the accurate identification of nerves during the course of surgical detection is critical to the success of the operation. Of course, further study is needed to evaluate the advantages of the use of this equipment as well as the cost. Could it, or a variant, also be used to show the potential long-term effects/success after nerve repair or nerve graft surgery?

S. H. Miller, MD

Neoplasms

Network geometry shows evidence sequestration for medical vs. surgical practices: treatments for basal cell carcinoma

Kim DD, Tang JY, Ioannidis JPA (Stanford Univ School of Medicine, Redwood City, CA; Stanford Prevention Res Ctr, CA)

J Clin Epidemiol 67:391-400, 2014

Objectives.—Basal cell carcinoma (BCC) is the most common cancer with 2 million treatments per year with little evidence-based guidelines for treatment. There are three classes of interventions (surgical, destructive, and topical) for BCC, and this study aimed to determine whether there are preferences or avoidances in comparisons of different types of treatments for BCC in randomized controlled trials (RCTs).

Study Design and Setting.—PubMed, Cochrane Central Registry of Clinical Trials, and ClinicalTrials.Gov were used to identify eligible published and registered ongoing RCTs.

Results.—Fifty-five trials (42 published and 13 registered trials) were identified. Only one unpublished registered trial compared a topical vs. a surgical intervention, and only one trial compared a topical vs. a destructive intervention. Conversely, 44 of the 55 trials compared interventions within the same treatment class and 9 of 55 trials compared surgical vs. destructive interventions. In most trials, selection of same-class comparators was not necessitated by the type of BCC lesions (nonaggressive superficial or nodular vs. aggressive, infiltrative, morpheic BCCs, $P = 0.155$) or their location (face vs. nonfacial, $P = 0.137$).

Conclusion.—This is the first time that an evaluation of network geometry is applied to address issues of comparisons between different families of interventions that belong to different specialties and practices (medical vs. surgical). Previous evaluations of homophily have addressed different families of interventions, in which all interventions are medical (drugs) and performed in the same health-care settings. The noncommunicating bodies of evidence between medical and surgical interventions that we document highlight a problem of unnecessary sequestration of the evidence and the corresponding health-care practices.

▶ This article is the first time an evaluation of network geometry has been applied to address issues of comparisons among different families of interventions that belong to different specialties and practices (medical vs surgical). This emphasizes that noncommunicating bodies of evidence between medical and surgical interventions highlight a problem of unnecessary sequestration of evidence and the corresponding health care practices. This article introduces new concepts such as trial networks to compare treatments. This is a totally different way to evaluate treatments and is important in that it compares medical and surgical treatments.

D. J. Smith, Jr, MD

Head & Neck Reconstruction

Development of the Pectoral Perforator Flap and the Deltopectoral Perforator Flap Pedicled With the Pectoralis Major Muscle Flap

Nishi Y, Rikimaru H, Kiyokawa K, et al (Kurume Univ School of Medicine, Fukuoka, Japan)

Ann Plast Surg 71:365-371, 2013

Purpose.—Because thinning of the pectoralis major myocutaneous flap is impossible due to blood circulation, it is difficult to produce thin flaps. Although the pectoral flap and the deltopectoral flap are the best flaps that provide a highly desirable color-texture match to facial skin, their reach is restricted and they require resection in 2 stages. The purpose of this paper is to develop a new method of elevating a flap and to resolve these problems.

Methods.—First, include the third intercostal perforating branch of the internal thoracic artery in the skin paddle and, outward therefrom, design a skin paddle of the pectoral flap in accordance with the shape of the defect. After a skin incision along the design, elevate the pectoral flap pedicled with the third intercostal perforating branch. Then, after cutting the third intercostal perforating branch at the lower surface of the pectoralis major muscle, harvest the approximately 5- to 6-cm-wide pectoralis

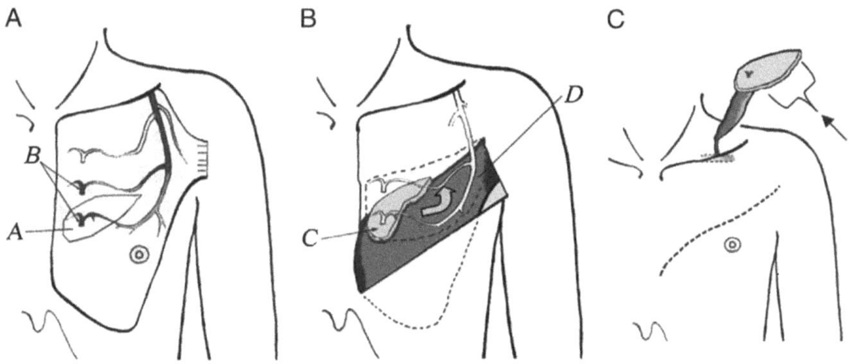

FIGURE 3.—Method of elevating the pectoral perforator flap and the DP perforator flap. A, Design of the pectoral perforator flap. *A*, Design the skin paddle in accord with the defective region. *B*, Include the second and third intercostal perforating branches of the internal thoracic artery. B, Method of elevating the pectoral perforator flap and DP perforator flap pedicled with the pectoralis major myocutaneous flap. *C*, Skin paddle of the elevated pectoral perforator flap (yellow arrow). *D*, Range for harvesting the muscle body of the pectoralis major muscle (blue broken line). The muscle body of the pectoralis major muscle (black broken line), including the muscular branch of the second and third intercostal branches and the pectoral branch of the thoracoacromial artery, is harvested laterally. C, Pectoral perforator flap after elevation. The skin paddle and the muscle body of the pectoralis major muscle are consolidated only in the part of their perforating branches and, by detaching the skin paddle from the muscle body, the reach of the flap is extended on a pro rata basis (arrow). The donor site is sutured at a single time. For Interpretation of the references to color in this figure legend, the reader is referred to web version of this article. (Reprinted from Nishi Y, Rikimaru H, Kiyokawa K, et al. Development of the pectoral perforator flap and the deltopectoral perforator flap pedicled with the pectoralis major muscle flap. *Ann Plast Surg*. 2013;71:365-371, with permission from Lippincott Williams & Wilkins.)

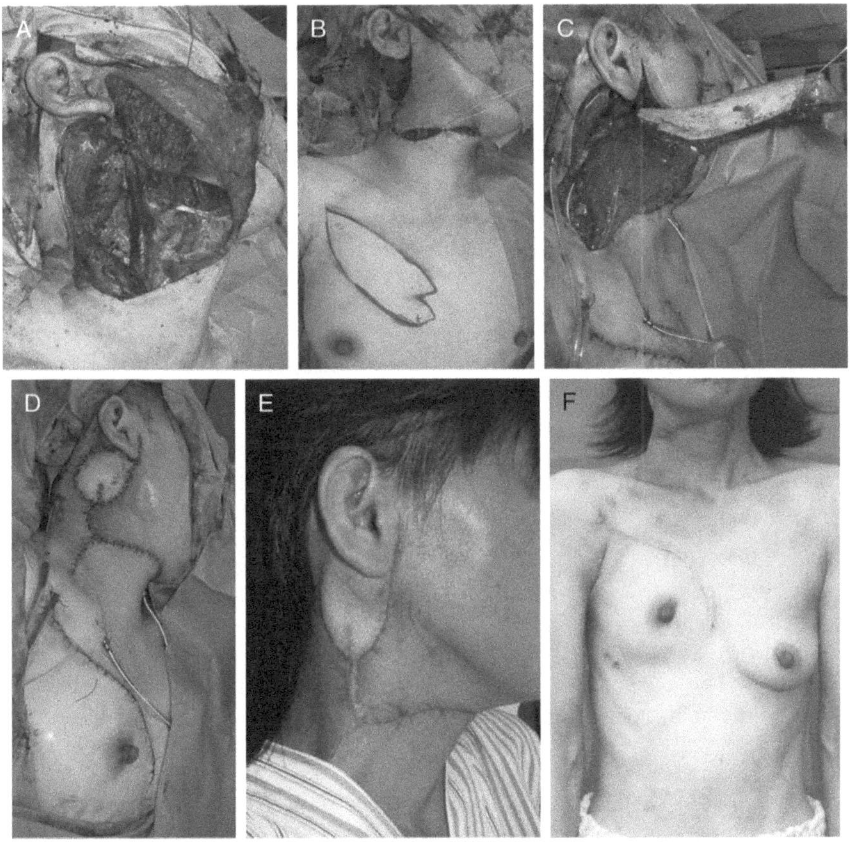

FIGURE 5.—Case 2. A 54-year-old woman who underwent total resection of the right parotid gland—skin defects in the lower portion of the right pinna. A, Findings immediately after total resection of the parotid gland. The carotid artery is exposed by neck dissection. B, The defect range of the lower right ear and the design of the pectoral perforator flap. C, The pectoral perforator flap pedicled with the pectoralis major muscle flap is elevated and moved to the neck region. D, Findings immediately after surgery. The donor site is sutured at a single time. E, Findings at 2 months after surgery. The flap is completely grafted. F, Findings of the donor site at 2 months after surgery. (Reprinted from Nishi Y, Rikimaru H, Kiyokawa K, et al. Development of the pectoral perforator flap and the deltopectoral perforator flap pedicled with the pectoralis major muscle flap. *Ann Plast Surg*. 2013;71:365-371, with permission from Lippincott Williams & Wilkins.)

major muscle in the lateral direction. In doing so, it is important to include in the harvested muscle body of the pectoralis major muscle the muscular branch of the third intercostal perforating branch, the branch of thoracoacromial artery, as well as the true anastomosis of both. Thereafter, elevate the entire flap, with the thoracoacromial artery for vascularization, and move it to the head and neck region via the subclavian route. In this way, the pectoral perforator flap pedicled with the pectoralis major muscle flap (PP flap) is elevated. As for the deltopectoral perforator flap with the pectoralis major muscle flap (DPP flap), after elevating the deltopectoral flap pedicled with both the second and third intercostal perforating branches of the internal thoracic artery, carry out the same flap elevation operations.

Results.—The PP flap was used in 4 cases and the DPP flap was used in 1 case. In all cases, the flaps were completely grafted and quite satisfactory, functional, as well as demonstrating good cosmetic results.

Discussion.—Unlike the conventional pectoralis major myocutaneous flap, the PP flap does not contain in its skin paddle the pectoralis major muscle and the mammary gland, making it possible to produce a thin flap. In addition, the development of this method has now substantially extended the reach of the flap, thereby making it possible for the PP flap to reach the oropharyngeal region and for the DPP flap to reach the frontal region at a single time. Originally, the skin over the precordium is relatively thin and flexible and provides a desirable color-texture match to facial and neck skin; therefore, it is believed that this method may serve as an extremely useful means in the future in the functional and cosmetic reconstruction of the head and neck region (Figs 3 and 5).

▶ Better understanding and detailed delineation of the vascular anatomy of circulation within the pectoralis major myocutaneous flap have allowed the authors to develop relatively thinner flaps for head and neck reconstruction than was possible using standard pectoralis myocutaneous flaps and deltopectoral flaps. The key to their success lies in the practical demonstration of the anastomotic relationship between the major blood supply to the pectoralis major muscle, the thoracoacromial artery, and the second and third intercostal perforating branches of the internal thoracic artery, which are the primary blood supplies to the deltopectoral flap within the body of the pectoralis major muscle.[1] They reported 100% success in 7 patients, 6 in which the pectoralis major flap was used and one in which a deltopectoral flap was used. The authors propose that these flaps are useful alternatives for reconstruction when microsurgery is not available. Several drawbacks remain obvious. One is that if the deltopectoral flap is used, closure of the donor site requires a 2-stage procedure or a skin grafted donor site, and both of these flaps do distort the female breast.

S. H. Miller, MD

Reference

1. Rikimaru H, Kiyokawa K, Inoue Y, et al. Three-dimensional anatomical vascular distribution in the pectoralis major myocutaneous flap. *Plast Reconstr Surg*. 2005; 11:1342-1352.

Lymphedema

Prospective, randomized, controlled trial comparing the effectiveness of adjustable compression Velcro wraps versus inelastic multicomponent compression bandages in the initial treatment of leg lymphedema

Damstra RJ, Partsch H (Nij Smellinghe Hosp, Drachten, The Netherlands; Univ of Vienna, Austria)

J Vasc Surg Venous Lymphat Disord 1:13-19, 2013

Background.—Inelastic multicomponent compression (ICM) bandages applied by specialized medical staff are the standard of care for compression therapy of lymphedema of the extremities. However, new adjustable compression wraps (ACWs), which can be applied by patients themselves and, up to now, have been mainly recommended for the maintenance treatment phase of lymphedema, may be an important step toward the self-management of the initial treatment phase.

Methods.—This prospective, randomized, controlled comparative study assessed the effectiveness of an ACW in the treatment of leg lymphedema, compared with the traditional treatment with conventional IMC bandages. Included were 30 hospitalized patients admitted due to moderate to severe unilateral lymphedema (stages 2-3) of the leg. The primary outcome measures in both groups were reduction in volume of the affected leg and interface pressure after 2 and 24 hours. Patients were randomized into two groups of 15 patients: group A received ACW and group B received IMC bandages, both applied by experienced staff. After 2 hours, the staff replaced IMC bandages and the patients applied ACW, as previously instructed. Finally, compression was removed after 24 hours. Classic water displacement volumetry was performed before compression and after 2 hours and after 24 hours of compression. The interface pressure was measured immediately after application of compression, 2 hours after compression, before and after compression renewal, and finally, after 24 hours. Patients in the ACW group were allowed to adjust the wrap themselves when they considered it necessary.

Results.—The reduction in median volume after 2 hours was 109 mL (interquartile range [IQR], 64–271 mL; −3.1%) in the ACW group and 75 mL (IQR, 41–135; −2.4%) in the IMC group (not significant). After 24 hours, the reduction in median volume was 339 mL (IQR, 231–493 mL; −10.3%) in the ACW group and 190 mL (IQR, 113–296 mL; −5.9%) in the IMC group ($P < .05$). The interface pressure dropped significantly after 2 and 24 hours in the IMC group (−50% and −6%), but significantly less in the ACW group (−26% and −44%), mainly due to self-readjustment. The median pressures achieved after self-application of ACW (52 mm Hg; IQR, 44–61 mm Hg) were of the same order as those produced by the nurses after the first application of ACW (53 mm Hg; IQR, 39–59 mm Hg), with less variation.

Conclusions.—In patients with moderate to severe lymphedema of the legs, ACW achieved a significantly more pronounced reduction in volume after 24 hours than IMC bandages. Patients were able to apply and adjust the device after being instructed in its use and after an initial 2-hour period of wear. Autonomous handling of ACW seemed to improve the clinical outcome and is a promising step toward self-management involving effective compression.

► Plastic surgeons caring for patients with lymphedema of the upper or lower extremity should be apprised of the newer recommendations of the International Compression Club regarding the 4 central properties of compression bandages, P-LA-C-E: pressure, layers, compression, and elasticity. In this prospective, albeit small, study with limited power, the authors showed that the outcomes for patient-adjustable compression Velcro wraps were statistically superior to those of professionally applied inelastic multicomponent compression bandages (IMC) in the initial treatment of leg lymphedema. Potential concerns with the conclusion in this preliminary study, in addition to the limited power, include nonblinding of the observers as to treatment techniques, short study time, and differences in the 2 groups regarding primary vs secondary lymphedema. Nonetheless, this patient-entered technology does have promise providing a cost-benefit analysis can also show its efficacy and efficiency when compared with IMC.

S. H. Miller, MD

A Prospective Analysis of 100 Consecutive Lymphovenous Bypass Cases for Treatment of Extremity Lymphedema

Chang DW, Suami H, Skoracki R (Univ of Texas M. D. Anderson Cancer Ctr, Houston)

Plast Reconstr Surg 132:1305-1314, 2013

Background.—The authors prospectively evaluated the efficacy of lymphovenous bypass in patients with lymphedema secondary to cancer treatment.

Methods.—The authors prospectively enrolled 100 consecutive patients with extremity lymphedema secondary to cancer treatment. Sixty-five patients underwent lymphovenous bypass with indocyanine green fluorescent lymphangiography. Evaluation included qualitative assessment and quantitative volumetric analysis before and 3, 6, and 12 months after bypass.

Results.—Lymphovenous bypass was performed in 89 upper extremities and 11 lower extremities. For upper extremity lymphedemas, the mean preoperative volume differential was 32 percent. Symptom improvement was reported by 96 percent of patients and quantitative improvement was noted by 74 percent. The overall mean volume differential reduction was 33 percent at 3 months, 36 percent at 6 months, and 42 percent at 12 months after surgery. The mean volume differential reductions at 3, 6, and 12 months after lymphovenous bypass in patients with stage 1 or 2 lymphedema (58, 52, and 61 percent, respectively) were significantly larger than those in the patients with stage 3 or 4 lymphedema (12, 16, and 17 percent, respectively). Eleven bypasses were performed in seven patients with lower extremity lymphedema, with a mean preoperative volume differential of 38 percent. Only four (57 percent) of these patients reported symptom improvement; postoperative volume measurements were available for only two of these four.

Conclusions.—Lymphovenous bypass can be effective in reducing lymphedema severity, particularly in patients with early-stage upper extremity lymphedema. Indocyanine green lymphangiography accurately identified functional lymphatic vessels and may have a role in objectively assessing lymphedema severity and patient selection.

Clinical Question/Level of Evidence.—Therapeutic, IV.

▶ This is an early prospective article reporting the types of preoperative and postoperative study as well as outcomes of a mixed bag of patients with postoperative lymphedema of the upper and lower extremity treated at the MD Anderson Hospital. Although the study reports on 100 patients, in fact, the first 35 were not studied using indocyanine green fluorescent lymphangiography. It is fairly obvious that the latter is an excellent state-of-the art technique to finding lymphatic vessels and to evaluate the severity of the lymphedema preoperatively. It is not surprising that the authors found that results in limbs less severely affected by lymphedema did better after the procedure than in those with more advanced disease, in which fewer lymphatics were available for anastomosis and the tissues tended to be more fibrotic and less amenable to volumetric reduction. It also seems obvious that lymphedema of the upper and lower extremity are quite different and best studied separately. I was intrigued by the potential for the development of a severity staging index as well as an index to assess outcomes based on using indocyanine green fluorescent lymphangiography. Further work is necessary if this is to come to fruition.

S. H. Miller, MD

Operative Treatment of Peripheral Lymphedema: A Systematic Meta-Analysis of the Efficacy and Safety of Lymphovenous Microsurgery and Tissue Transplantation

Basta MN, Gao LL, Wu LC (Perelman School of Medicine at the Univ of Pennsylvania, Philadelphia; Hosp of the Univ of Pennsylvania, Philadelphia; Univ of Pennsylvania Health Systems, Philadelphia)

Plast Reconstr Surg 133:905-913, 2014

Background.—The purpose of this study was to quantify the efficacy and safety of microsurgery for lymphedema through a systematic meta-analysis, which has not been described before.

Methods.—A literature search was conducted to identify all articles involving microsurgical treatment of lymphedema. Studies meeting criteria for inclusion were rated on methodologic quality based on the American Society of Plastic Surgeons levels of evidence. Demographic information, cause of lymphedema, and surgical technique were recorded. Quantitative change in lymphedema and perioperative complications were noted.

Results.—Twenty-seven studies were included, with 24 offering level IV evidence and three offering level III evidence. Lymphovenous shunt procedures were performed in 22 studies and lymph node transplantation was performed in five. Excess circumference was reduced by 48.8 ± 6.0 percent, and absolute circumference was reduced by 3.31 ± 0.73 cm. Studies reporting change in volume demonstrated reduction in excess volume by 56.6 ± 9.1 percent, and absolute volume was reduced by 23.6 ± 2.1 percent. The incidence of no improvement in lymphedema postoperatively was 11.8 percent, and 91.2 percent of patients reported subjective improvement. Approximately 64.8 percent of patients discontinued compression garments at follow-up. Complications included operative-site infection (4.7 percent), lymphorrhea (7.7 percent), reexploration for flap congestion (2.7 percent), and additional procedures (22.6 percent).

Conclusions.—Operative interventions for peripheral lymphedema appear to provide consistent quantitative improvements postoperatively, with a relatively wide safety margin. Lymph node transplantation may provide better outcomes compared with lymphovenous shunt, but well-designed head-to-head comparisons are needed to evaluate this further.

Clinical Question/Level of Evidence.—Therapeutic, III.

▶ The authors quantified the efficacy and safety of microsurgery in the treatment of lymphedema through a systematic meta-analysis. They concluded that operative interventions for peripheral lymphedema appear to provide consistent quantitative improvements postoperatively, with a relatively wide safety margin. Scanning the references shows that most of this work is done outside of the United States. I don't see a lot of enthusiasm nationally for doing this. I wonder why the international experience is so much more positive.

D. J. Smith, Jr, MD

Microsurgery for groin lymphocele and lymphedema after oncologic surgery

Boccardo F, Dessalvi S, Campisi C, et al (IRCCS S.Martino Univ Hosp—IST, Genoa, Italy)

Microsurgery 34:10-13, 2014

Groin lymphocele (GL) is a frequent complication of inguinal lymph node dissection, and conservative treatment is not always successful. Different surgical methods have been used to treat lymphoceles arising from lymphatics injured during groin surgery. However, they all involve the closure of lymphatics merging at the lymphocele, increasing the risk of postoperative lower limb lymphedema or of worsening lymphedema if already clinically evident. We assessed the efficacy of a diagnostic and therapeutic protocol to manage inguinal lymphoceles using lymphoscintigraphy (LS) and microsurgical procedures. Sixteen GL [seven associated with leg lymphedema (LL)] were studied by LS preoperatively and treated by complete excision of lymphocele and microsurgical lymphatic-venous anastomoses between afferent lymphatics and a collateral branch of great saphenous vein. Lower limb lymphatics were identified intraoperatively using Patent Blue dye injection. Nine patients without lymphedema had complete healing of lymphocele and no appearance of lower limb postoperative lymphedema. The other seven patients with associated secondary lymphedema had complete disappearance of lymphocele and a remarkable reduction of leg volume. Four of them completely recovered without the need of any compression garment, after the first year postoperative. Inguinal lymphocele nonresponsive to conservative treatment can be advantageously studied by LS and successfully treated by microsurgical reconstructive procedures, above all if associated to LL.

▶ The authors conclude that inguinal lymphoceles nonresponsive to conservative treatment can be advantageously studied by lymphoscintigraphy and successfully treated by microsurgical reconstructive procedures. The authors studied 16 patients. The 9 without lymphedema had complete healing of the lymphocele and no lower extremity edema. More impressive are the 7 patients with associated secondary lymphedema. Not only did they have complete resolution of their lymphocele, but they also had significant reduction in their lymphedema. Four completely recovered with no need for compression garments. Historically, a microsurgical approach to these problems has not done well. Increasingly, there are reports of success transfer or microsurgical drainage. Perhaps it is time to reassess this entire area.

D. J. Smith, Jr, MD

3 Trauma

Head and Neck

Still no reliable consensus in management of blow-out fracture

Alinasab B, Ryott M, Stjärne P (Karolinska Univ Hosp, Stockholm, Sweden)

Injury 45:197-202, 2014

Background.—Management of blow-out fractures (BOF) is addressed by different specialties. The general agreement is that patients with the potential for late enophthalmus development require early surgical intervention. In this study we wanted to: (i) evaluate the differences in opinions between the specialties that manage BOF and also whether there was a difference between surgeons from different countries, (ii) evaluate if surgeons handle these cases based upon their own individual criteria, (iii) evaluate the correlation between the management of patients with orbital floor fractures and any late sequelae detected upon eye examination.

Materials and Methods.—Eleven patients with BOF were selected from the records of the Department of ENT and Head & Neck Surgery, Karolinska University Hospital between 2003 and 2008. The cases were presented with a case history and CT scans to 46 surgeons from different countries and specialties and they were asked to give their opinions regarding the need for surgery, timing of surgery and the risk for late enophthalmus. We considered a group of surgeons to be in agreement if there was ≥75% agreement on whether or not to operate, when to operate and on the risk for late enophthalmus.

Result.—The surgeons agreed on the choice of management for the patients (whether or not to operate) in only 5 of the 11 cases. Similarly, in only 5 of the 11 cases did the surgeons agree upon the risk for late enophthalmus. There was a greater difference between specialities than between physicians from the participating countries.

Conclusion.—There are considerable differences in opinions regarding the management of BOF due to a lack of a reliable consensus. The management of BOF appears to be based on both individual and local traditions. Guidelines based on a randomized prospective study in BOF are required.

▶ I believe this to be a very valuable study that may act as a model to stimulate other such studies wherein there seems to be little consensus regarding need for treatment, timing of treatment, and consequences of treatment and nontreatment of blow-out fractures. It is unclear to me as to whether the material sent to the evaluating surgeons also consisted of photographs of the involved eye to show the degree of injury and its effect on the orbital contents. It is disconcerting to see the lack of agreement between different specialties and different countries. I clearly agree that further prospective studies are needed to establish more universal guidelines. I am interested in the author's speculation about membership in the AO Foundation accounting for the high incidence of surgical intervention by the Swiss-German physicians resulting in a more unified approach to the problem.

S. H. Miller, MD

Orbital fractures in children: A review of outcomes

Gerber B, Kiwanuka P, Dhariwal D (Northampton General Hosp, UK; The Royal London Hosp, London, UK; John Radcliffe Hosp, Headington, Oxford, UK)
Br J Oral Maxillofac Surg 51:789-793, 2013

The third most common facial fractures in children are fractures of the orbit, and the medial wall and floor are the commonest sites affected. The aetiology, clinical presentation, and timing of operation all differ from those of adults. If there are few or no clinical signs, but oculocardiac reflex is present, it is highly suggestive of trapdoor injury. This retrospective study includes all consecutive children (younger than 18 years) referred with confirmed fractures of the orbital floor over a 5-year period (2005–2010). A total of 24 patients were identified with a mean age of 13.5 years, and most injuries were secondary to falls. Isolated injury to the orbital floor occurred in 14 (58%); the rest involved other fractures of the orbital wall or face, or both. There were 11 trapdoor fractures (46%), and 9 open blow-out fractures (38%). Overall, nausea and vomiting occurred in 13 patients (54%); 8 of these had trapdoor fractures. Most patients had operations (22, 92%), and the mean time to operation was 4 days. Complications increased with delays to theatre. Those operated on within 1 day had fewer complications than those who had operations after 3 days. Postoperatively, diplopia ($n = 6/11$) and restricted eye movement ($n = 3/11$) were associated with trapdoor injury, while enophthalmos ($n = 1/9$) and paraesthesia ($n = 3/9$) were related to open blow-out fractures. To reduce compromised outcomes, prompt operation is warranted in all children with fractures of the orbital floor regardless of the configuration.

▶ Periorbital fractures are ubiquitous in the practice of most plastic surgeons who participate in trauma call, and the signs and symptoms of these injuries are generally well known. Less common are orbital fractures in children, especially those less than 14 years of age, and the causes, presentations, and timing of surgical procedures. Trapdoor injuries in children are common, likely caused by a "greenstick" fracture of the orbital floor and subsequent trapdoor effect of the orbital contents. Children also are likely to have nausea and vomiting with these injuries, and that should heighten the clinician's suspicion. Furthermore, delays in freeing up the tissue trapped does result in poorer outcomes, and thus early treatment is mandatory.

S. H. Miller, MD

Extremities and Trunk

The Flexor Digitorum Longus Muscle Flap for the Reconstruction of Soft-Tissue Defects in the Distal Third of the Leg: Anatomic Considerations and Clinical Applications

Durand S, Sita-Alb L, Ang S, et al (Hospital Avicenne, Bobigny, France; Inst of Anatomy, Paris, France)

Ann Plast Surg 71:595-599, 2013

Soft-tissue defects of the distal third of the leg are common occurrences in trauma centers. The authors present the anatomic basis and their clinical experience using the flexor digitorum longus muscle flap. Ten cadaver specimens were dissected to evaluate the potential use of this flap for soft-tissue coverage in the lower third of the leg. Eleven patients underwent a soft-tissue reconstruction in the distal third of the leg with this flap. The average size of the defect covered by this flap was 11.3 cm^2. This transfer flap was used in 7 cases exclusively or in combination in 4 cases. No functional deficit and good plastic result were observed in all cases. Ease of elevation and reliability has made this transfer flap the procedure of choice for small soft-tissue defects over the proximal portion of the distal tibia in our institution.

► This is a review of a flap well described by others[1] but further elucidated by these authors. The ease of dissection and minimal, if any, donor site or functional deformity are positive attributes, but the size of the defects that can be covered is quite limited. In this study, the primary flexor digitorum longus flap had to be combined with a portion of the soleus muscle or a combination of the soleus and gastrocnemius in 4 of 11 cases. Defects of the distal third of the leg are notoriously difficult to cover, and various muscles, fasciocutaneous flaps, and distally based flaps have all been reported to be useful in small studies. What is lacking is a more comprehensive report with documentation of which flaps are most useful when faced with distal third defects of the lower extremity of varying size and when none are likely to be as successful as the more difficult and time-consuming free flap. The authors' stress on the need for preoperative study of the vascularity of the lower limb is well taken as is their cautious note about using this flap in older patients with secondary morbidity, especially that involving vasculature.

S. H. Miller, MD

Reference

1. Mathes SJ, Nahai F. *Reconstructive Surgery: Principles, Anatomy and Technique.* New York, NY: Churchill Livingstone, Inc; 1997. 1371–1380.

Burns

An Open, Prospective, Randomized Pilot Investigation Evaluating Pain With the Use of a Soft Silicone Wound Contact Layer Vs Bridal Veil and Staples on Split Thickness Skin Grafts as a Primary Dressing

Patton ML, Mullins RF, Smith D, et al (Crozer-Chester Med Ctr, Upland, PA; Joseph M. Still Res Foundation, Inc, Augusta, GA; Florida Gulf-to-Bay Anesthesiology, Tampa; et al)
J Burn Care Res 34:674-681, 2013

An open, prospective, randomized, pilot investigation was implemented to evaluate the pain, cost-effectiveness, ease of use, tolerance, efficacy, and safety of a soft silicone wound contact layer (Mepitel® One) vs Bridal Veil and staples used on split thickness skin grafts in the treatment of deep partial or full-thickness thermal burns. Individuals aged between 18 and 70 years with deep partial or full-thickness thermal burns (1–25% TBSA) were randomized into two groups and treated for 14 days or until greater than 95% graft take was achieved, whichever occurred first. Data were obtained and analyzed on pain experienced before, during, and after dressing removal. Secondary considerations included the overall cost (direct), graft take and healing, the ease of product use, overall experience of the dressing, and adverse events. A total of 43 subjects were recruited. There were no significant differences in burn area profiles within the groups. The pain level during dressing removal was significant between the groups (P =.0118) with the removal of Mepitel One being less painful. The staff costs were lower in the group of patients treated with Mepitel One (P =.0064) as reflected in the shorter time required for dressing removal (P =.0005), with Mepitel One taking on average less than a quarter of the time to remove. There was no significant difference in healing between the two groups, with 99.0% of the Mepitel One group and 93.1% of the Bridal Veil and staples group showing greater than 95% graft take at post-op day 7 (+/−1) (P =.2373). Clinicians reported that the soft silicone dressing was easier to use, more conformable, and demonstrated better ability to stay in place, compared with the Bridal Veil and staples regime. Both treatments were well tolerated, with no serious adverse events in either treatment group. Mepitel One was at least as effective in the treatment of patients as the standard care (Bridal Veil and staples). In addition, the group of patients treated with the soft silicone dressing demonstrated decreased pain and lower costs associated with treatment.

▶ This is a worthwhile initial prospective, multicentered, randomized, pilot study investigating 2 types of post–skin graft dressings used after treatment of partial or full-thickness burn wounds. One must ask these authors to explain the reasons for the choice of the 2 types of dressings, soft silicone (Mepitel One) and bridal veil as opposed to other materials in common use. One might also question whether some of the differences, at least in the assessment of pain during dressing changes, were due, at least in part, to the use of staples holding the bridal veil in place rather than using sutures. I am uncertain that the data regarding costs, reported as total costs, really took into account the costs of the material used and the labor costs required to change the dressings. The grafts were meshed at 1:1 and 3:1 ratios, but it is unclear if the ratios for the meshed grafts were similar in the 2 treatment groups. Further work from this multicenter group should focus on larger groups, with adequate power to assess differences, longer-term follow-up, and quality of the healed graft.

S. H. Miller, MD

Cost study of dermal substitutes and topical negative pressure in the surgical treatment of burns

Hop MJ, TOPSKIN Study Group (Maasstad Hosp, Rotterdam, The Netherlands; et al)

Burns 40:388-396, 2014

Background.—A recently performed randomised controlled trial investigated the clinical effectiveness of dermal substitutes (DS) and split skin grafts (SSG) in combination with topical negative pressure (TNP) in the surgical treatment of burn wounds. In the current study, medical and non-medical costs were investigated, to comprehensively assess the benefits of this new treatment.

Methods.—The primary outcome was mean total costs of the four treatment strategies: SSG with or without DS, and with or without TNP. Costs were studied from a societal perspective. Findings were evaluated in light of the clinical effects on scar elasticity.

Results.—Eighty-six patients were included. Twelve months postoperatively, highest elasticity was measured in scars treated with DS and TNP ($p = 0.027$). The initial cost price of treatment with DS and TNP was €2912 compared to treatment with SSG alone €1703 ($p < 0.001$). However, mean total costs per patient did not differ significantly between groups (range €29 097–€43 774).

Discussion.—Costs of the interventional treatment contributed maximal 7% to the total costs and total costs varied widely within and between groups, but were not significantly different. Therefore, in the selection of the most optimal type of surgical intervention, cost considerations should not play an important role.

▶ This is a very interesting small ($n = 86$) randomized control study comparing the costs of burn wound treatment in 4 groups. In 1 arm, the authors used dermal substitutes (DS), split thickness (SS) mesh grafts, and topical negative pressure (TNP); in another arm, they used split thickness mesh grafts alone; in another group, they use split thickness meshed grafts and dermal substitute; and in the final arm, split thickness meshed skin grafts and topical negative pressure were used. The study was performed in 3 Dutch centers and assessed the cost-effectiveness of the treatments. It is unclear as to whether the meshed grafts were uniform at the 3 centers. The authors concluded that the optimal surgical treatment

(SS, DS, and TNP), at least as regards to measured scar elasticity, at 12 months did not cost more in total patient costs. Intervention costs were higher by 7% in the SS, DS, and TNP) group, but they amounted to a small percentage of the total patient care costs for the year. This study is a good start, but more patients are needed, and patients with third-degree burn wounds larger than 1% to 2% total body surface area need to be included. Finally, long-term benefits evaluating more than just elasticity of the healed wounds need to be assessed beyond the 12 months reported in this study. Ultimately, it remains to be seen if this combination therapy will limit the need for ongoing and long-term therapy, surgical and nonsurgical, for burn patients. That will be the true measure of its cost-effectiveness.

S. H. Miller, MD

4 Hand and Upper Extremity

Extremity

What's New in Hand Surgery

Amadio PC (Mayo Clinic, Rochester, MN)

J Bone Joint Surg Am 95:570-574, 2013

Background.—An update on the latest advances in hand surgery was done, using material presented at the annual meetings of the American Society for Surgery of the Hand, American Association for Hand Surgery, and American Academy of Orthopaedic Surgeons plus articles on hand surgery published between August 2011 and July 2012.

Skeletal Trauma.—Wrist fractures are usually managed surgically, but studies support the use of nonoperative treatment as well. Surgery may improve radiographic appearance but not necessarily function, causes higher rates of complications, and can require further surgery. Currently internal fixation costs $3516 whereas casting costs just 564. Patients may prefer surgery slightly more than casting, but the difference is not sufficient to outweigh the cost fact. Surgery for scaphoid fractures allows a quicker return to function and a lower nonunion rate, but more complications than casting. Both achieve similar final outcomes, pain experiences, and patient satisfaction levels. However, casting of displaced fractures has an 18% rate of nonunion compared to about 1% with surgery. If the proximal pole is involved, nonunion with casting may reach 34%, so surgery may be a better choice for displaced scaphoid fractures. For undisplaced fractures, the morbidity associated with casting depends on elbow and thumb immobilization. If computed tomography (CT) is used to assess displacement, union rates are significantly higher for patients who wear below-the-elbow casts excluding the thumb.

Dupuytren Contracture.—Collagenase may be effective for Dupuytren disease, especially at the metacarpophalangeal joint but may not be as cost-effective as open partial fasciectomy. The cost of collagenase per quality-adjusted life year (QALY) may be as high as $166,000. Open surgery cost is less likely to be accompanied by recurrence than needle aponeurotomy plus collagenase (21% versus 85%). Patient satisfaction levels are high, but patients tend to prefer the needle procedure even with the risk of recurrence because it offers a fast recovery, fewer complications, and minimal invasiveness.

Nerve.—When patients with carpal tunnel syndrome have severe thenar muscle atrophy and no motor conduction on electrodiagnostic tests, the surgeon must decide whether to do a tendon transfer immediately or wait for possible motor recovery after carpal tunnel release. Patients younger than age 50 years are more likely to see recovery, whereas those who are older have a chance of spontaneous recovery of about 50%. Nerve conduits are often preferred to nerve grafts. Length of the gap affects outcomes for processed allografts, with about half of those with gaps less than 15 mm having a return of good muscle strength and some two-point discrimination; a third of patients with gaps of 15 to 29 mm having sensory recovery, although motor recovery remains good; and few patients recovering sensory or motor recovery with gaps between 30 and 50 mm.

Arthritis.—Thumb carpometacarpal arthritis is more common in women than men. The latest hypothesis for causation suggests a role for the hormone relaxin. It relaxes pelvic ligaments before childbirth but also enhances sperm motility. Relaxin receptors are in the thumb carpometacarpal ligaments of both men and women, but considerably more are found in women. Based on these numbers, relaxin may influence thumb carpometacarpal ligament function and explain women's instability and thumb arthritis. Findings also suggest that silicone metacarpopholangeal joint arthroplasty may improve intermediate results in patients with rheumatoid arthritis, but the effects vanish after 3 years or so. Candidates for proximal interphalangeal joint arthroplasty may be managed with various options, including traditional silicone devices and newer metal and plastic or pyrocarbon implants. Over a mean of 3 years no lasting significant improvement in motion occurred, although the titanium/polyethylene and pyrocarbon devices achieved early improvement. All devices relieved pain. Surgical failure rates differed, with 2 of 18 silicone implants, 7 of 26 titanium/polyethylene implants, and 7 of 18 pyrocarbon implants requiring removal. Reasons for reoperation included extensor mechanism failure, collateral ligament instability, and joint contracture. The newer devices provide results that are different from but not necessarily better than those with silicone implants. Long-term study of a distal ulnar prosthesis to treat distal radioulnar joint instability found stable results for up to 11 years postoperatively. A linked distal radioulnar joint replacement arthroplasty used for 3 years showed improvement in 18 of 20 patients.

Kienböck Disease.—With early-stage involvement, revascularization or osteotomies to redistribute the load across the wrist may be helpful, but wrist arthrodesis is required for severe osseous collapse. If the lunate collapses and carpal malalignment develops without arthritis, midcarpal arthrodesis can correct the malalignment and unload the lunate. Scaphocapitate arthrodesis improves wrist motion, increases grip strength, and relieves pain effectively but also causes major complications.

Antibiotics, Follow-up, and Antiplatelet Medications.—A recent study of over 8000 consecutive clean elective hand surgery procedures found a low risk of infection, so antibiotics are not routinely indicated. Infection risk increases with smoking, diabetes, and longer procedures, but antibiotics are not protective against infection in these cases.

Postoperative follow-up after hand surgery is a consideration based on new health care management systems. In the United Kingdom, patients are followed for 3 months by the hand therapist and referred to the surgeon only if needed. This policy allows hand surgeons to focus on new patients and is less inconvenient for patients.

The advantages of continuing antiplatelet therapy appear to outweigh its disadvantages. A study of 76 patients who continued their antiplatelet drugs and 76 controls found no differences between groups in terms of pain, swelling, ecchymosis, or other postoperative measures.

Hand Surgery Education.—Currently the US model for hand surgery training requires a 1-year fellowship after training in orthopedic surgery, plastic surgery, or general surgery. A survey of hand directors found 65% supported the 1-year program, but 24% suggested a 5- or 6-year residence program in hand surgery. Nearly all believed training should be added in the care of wrist problems and peripheral nerve surgery. Less than half believed proficiency in microsurgery was needed, and less than a third supported burn, shoulder, elbow, or brachial plexus proficiency as a goal of the hand fellowship. In contrast, a survey of hand fellows trained between 2008 and 2010 found these fellows felt less comfortable with proximal arm problems, microsurgery, and brachial plexus care. Sixty percent said they would have applied for a 2-year fellowship if one were offered. A test of retention for a tendon repair teaching program found that more efforts will be needed to develop methods that produce a consistent grasp of previously learned skills.

▶ Dr Peter Amadio presents the Specialty Update for What's New in Hand Surgery. He covers skeletal trauma, Dupuytren contracture, nerve, arthritis, Kienböck disease, cost effectiveness of hand surgery, and education in hand surgery. Dr Amadio does a superb job of synthesizing and presenting his information. This is an excellent review.

D. J. Smith, Jr, MD

The Art and Science of Photography in Hand Surgery

Wang K, Kowalski EJ, Chung KC (Peking Union Med College, Beijing, China; Univ of Michigan Health System, Ann Arbor)

J Hand Surg Am 39:580-588, 2014

High-quality medical photography plays an important role in teaching and demonstrating the functional capacity of the hands as well as in medicolegal documentation. Obtaining standardized, high-quality photographs is now an essential component of many surgery practices. The importance of standardized photography in facial and cosmetic surgery has been well documented in previous studies, but no studies have thoroughly addressed the details of photography for hand surgery. In this paper, we provide a set of guidelines and basic camera concepts for different scenarios to help hand surgeons obtain appropriate and informative high-quality photographs. A camera used for medical photography should come equipped with a large sensor size and an optical zoom lens with a focal length ranging anywhere from 14 to 75 mm. In a clinic or office setting, we recommend 6 standardized views of the hand and 4 views for the wrist; additional views should be taken for tendon ruptures, nerve injuries, or other deformities of the hand. For intraoperative pictures, the camera operator should understand the procedure and pertinent anatomy in order to properly obtain high-quality photographs. When digital radiographs are not available and radiographic film must be photographed, it is recommended to reduce the exposure and change the color mode to black and white to obtain the best possible pictures. The goal of medical photography is to present the subject in an accurate and precise fashion.

▶ High-quality medical photography plays an important role in teaching and medicolegal documentation. For hand surgery, it can also demonstrate functional capacity. The authors provide guidelines for obtaining these photos. This is important because it standardizes the views and allows for more accurate comparison. For anyone not routinely using photography, this is a must. For those using it, the article provides a nice review.

D. J. Smith, Jr, MD

Essential Hand Surgery Procedures for Mastery by Graduating Plastic Surgery Residents: A Survey of Program Directors

Noland SS, Fischer LH, Lee GK, et al (Stanford Univ Hosp, CA; Univ of Washington Med Ctr, Seattle)

Plast Reconstr Surg 132:977e-984e, 2013

Background.—This study was designed to establish the essential hand surgery procedures that should be mastered by graduating plastic surgery residents. This framework can then be used as a guideline for developing Objective Structured Assessment of Technical Skill to teach technical skills in hand surgery.

Methods.—Ten expert hand surgeons were surveyed regarding the essential hand surgery procedures that should be mastered by graduating plastic surgery residents. The top 10 procedures from this survey were then used to survey all 89 Accreditation Council for Graduate Medical Education–approved plastic surgery program directors.

Results.—There was a 69 percent response rate to the program director survey ($n = 61$). The top nine hand surgery procedures included open carpal tunnel release, open A1 pulley release, digital nerve repair with microscope, closed reduction and percutaneous pinning of metacarpal fracture, excision of dorsal or volar ganglion, zone II flexor tendon repair with multistrand technique, incision and drainage of the flexor tendon sheath for flexor tenosynovitis, flexor tendon sheath steroid injection, and open cubital tunnel release.

Conclusions.—Surgical educators need to develop objective methods to teach and document technical skill. The Objective Structured Assessment of Technical Skill is a valid method for accomplishing this task. There has been no consensus regarding which hand surgery procedures should be mastered by graduating plastic surgery residents. The authors have identified nine procedures that are overwhelmingly supported by plastic surgery program directors. These nine procedures can be used as a guideline for developing Objective Structured Assessment of Technical Skill to teach and document technical skills in hand surgery.

▶ Within the Next Graduate Medical Education Accreditation System, surgical educators need to develop objective methods to teach and document technical skills. Through a survey of program directors, hand surgery procedures regarded as essential were identified and, therefore, necessary to be mastered by plastic surgery residents by the completion of their residency. This article is a must for anyone involved in residency training. Even for those not involved, it is a nice peek into the evolution of graduate training in plastic surgery.

D. J. Smith, Jr, MD

Evidence-Based Medicine: Metacarpal Fractures

Bloom JMP, Hammert WC (Univ of Rochester Med Ctr, NY)

Plast Reconstr Surg 133:1252-1260, 2014

Learning Objectives.—After studying this article, the participant should be able to: 1. Determine the need for operative treatment of metacarpal fractures. 2. Describe the position of immobilization for nonoperative treatment of fifth metacarpal fractures. 3. Assess the differences between intramedullary pinning and transverse pinning of displaced metacarpal fractures. 4. Compare the advantages of plating and pinning for treatment of displaced metacarpal fractures. 5. Recognize appropriate timing and treatment of open metacarpal fractures.

Summary.—The body of evidence regarding the treatment of metacarpal fractures continues to grow. Conservative management, closed reduction with percutaneous Kirschner wire fixation, intramedullary fixation, and open reduction and internal fixation with plates and/or screws are all accepted treatment modalities. The goal of this review is to highlight the most recent literature and the best evidence available for the management of metacarpal fractures.

▶ All of the Maintenance of Certification—continuing medical education articles have been excellent. These 4 (Evidence-Based Medicine: Dupuytren

Contracture, Evidence-Based Medicine: Flexor Tendon Repair, Evidence-Based Medicine: Metacarpal Fractures, Evidence-Based Medicine: Carpal Tunnel Syndrome) are no exception. The goal of the metacarpal fracture article, the flexor tendon article and the Dupuytren contracture article is to highlight the most recent literature and the best evidence available for the management of these 3 diseases. In the carpal tunnel syndrome article, Dr Lalonde concentrates on topics not covered in depth in the first 2 articles (first article 2008, summarization of best literature; second article, best evidence for assessment, surgical treatment, and outcomes from the literature published between 1999 and 2009) and provides an update of the highest level evidence on important topics between 2009 to 2013. All 4 articles achieve their goals admirably. Must read.

D. J. Smith, Jr, MD

Carpal Fractures

Suh N, Ek ET, Wolfe SW (Hosp for Special Surgery, NY; Monash Univ, Melbourne, Australia)

J Hand Surg Am 39:785-791, 2014

Carpal fractures are exceedingly rare clinical entities and are often associated with concomitant injuries. In this review, we focus on fractures of the carpus, excluding the scaphoid, and provide an update on the current consensus as to mechanism, diagnosis, management, outcomes, and complications after such injuries.

▶ Carpal fractures are rare clinical entities and often are associated with concomitant injuries. The authors provide the current concerns as to mechanism, diagnosis, management, outcomes, and complications of fractures of the carpus, excluding the scaphoid. This is a clear, concise review and an excellent overview for anyone doing this surgery.

D. J. Smith, Jr, MD

A Systematic Review of Distraction Osteogenesis in Hand Surgery: What Are the Benefits, Complication Rates, and Duration of Treatment?

Kempton SJ, McCarthy JE, Afifi AM (Univ of Wisconsin Hosp and Clinics, Madison)

Plast Reconstr Surg 133:1120-1130, 2014

Background.—This work analyzes the utility of distraction osteogenesis as a surgical option for the management of acquired and traumatic hand deformities through a systematic review of the published literature.

Methods.—A PubMed search for articles reporting results of distraction osteogenesis in the hand was performed. Data collected included age, sex, cause, bone distracted, latency period, distraction rate, consolidation period, treatment time, length gained, and complications. Proportion data variables were compared using the chi-square test. A meta-analysis was also performed to assess the size effect of variables on complication development.

Results.—Thirty articles (424 distractions) met inclusion criteria. The average length gained from distraction was 2.2 cm; the average total treatment time was 116 days; the average complication rate was 26.4 percent. Proportion analysis, including all articles, showed that congenital cause had significantly fewer complications compared with traumatic cause ($p = 0.0129$). A lower complication rate in pediatric patients compared with adults approached but did not reach significance ($p = 0.0507$). Studies that underwent meta-analysis, including only articles comparing both variables of interest, were homogeneous ($I^2 < 25$) and without publication bias (Kendall's tau $p > 0.05$ and symmetric funnel plot). None of the variables analyzed by meta-analysis had a significant odds ratio for complication development ($p > 0.05$).

Conclusion.—Despite distinct advantages, distraction osteogenesis is associated with a long duration of treatment and high complication rates, particularly in adults and in posttraumatic reconstruction.

Clinical Question/Level of Evidence.—Therapeutic, IV.

▶ These authors analyze the utility of distraction osteogenesis as a surgical option for the management of acquired and traumatic hand deformities through a systematic review of the literature. They found that although distinct advantages exist, distraction osteogenesis is associated with a long duration of treatment and high complication rates, particularly in adults and in posttraumatic reconstruction. Hand function was subjectively improved. This confirms a long-standing bias. Although the benefits are obvious, intense consultation with the patient is necessary before this long journey is started. An excellent review with numerous references. No prospective studies but statistical analysis shows that the studies included were homogeneous.

D. J. Smith, Jr, MD

Evidence-Based Medicine: Flexor Tendon Repair

Neumeister MW, Amalfi A, Neumeister E (Southern Illinois Univ School of Medicine, Springfield, IL)

Plast Reconstr Surg 133:1222-1233, 2014

Learning Objectives.—After studying this article, the participant should be able to: 1. Describe and apply the current evidence-based treatment of acute flexor tendon injuries. 2. Compare and contrast the current postoperative therapy regimens following repair of flexor tendons. 3. Apply an evidence-based decision-making process for suture techniques of flexor tendon injuries.

Summary.—Flexor tendon repair remains a challenge for hand surgeons to reliably obtain excellent results. Surgical decisions should rely on the surgeon's experience, outcome studies, and direct evidence. This review is a compilation of the evidence from the literature on optimizing outcomes for flexor tendon repair.

▶ All of the Maintenance of Certification—continuing medical education articles have been excellent. These 4 (Evidence-Based Medicine: Dupuytren Contracture, Evidence-Based Medicine: Flexor Tendon Repair, Evidence-Based Medicine: Metacarpal Fractures, Evidence-Based Medicine: Carpal Tunnel Syndrome) are no exception. The goal of the metacarpal fracture article, the flexor tendon article, and the Dupuytren contracture article is to highlight the most recent literature and the best evidence available for the management of these 3 diseases. In the carpal tunnel syndrome article, Dr Lalonde concentrates on topics not covered in depth in the first 2 articles (first article 2008, summarization of best literature; second article, best evidence for assessment, surgical treatment, and outcomes from the literature published between 1999 and 2009) and provides an update of the highest level evidence on important topics between 2009 to 2013. All 4 articles achieve their goals admirably. Must read.

D. J. Smith, Jr, MD

Flexor Tendon Repair, Rehabilitation, and Reconstruction

Sandvall BK, Kuhlman-Wood K, Recor C, et al (Univ of Washington, Seattle)

Plast Reconstr Surg 132:1493-1503, 2013

Background.—Flexor tendon injury is a common problem that plastic surgeons are called on to treat. Despite their common nature, they present a challenge, not necessarily in the surgical treatment per se but in the ability to achieve a "normal" finger as the end result. Because of the difficulty in attaining good outcomes, much continues to be studied and written about flexor tendon injury.

Methods.—The current literature on flexor tendon repair, rehabilitation, and reconstruction is reviewed.

Results.—Aspects reviewed include type of anesthesia, suture material and configuration, repairs in the different flexor tendon zones, types of tendon rehabilitation, complications of flexor tendon surgery, and flexor tendon reconstruction.

Conclusion.—This review provides an update on the current standards in the treatment of flexor tendon injury.

▶ The authors review the current literature on flexor tendon repair, rehabilitation, and reconstruction. They discuss the type of anesthesia, suture material and configuration, repairs in the different flexor tendon zones, types of tendon rehabilitation, complications, and flexor tendon reconstruction. This is an excellent, comprehensive, but concise, review of current standards in the treatment of flexor tendon injury.

D. J. Smith, Jr, MD

Peripheral Nerve Repair and Reconstruction

Griffin JW, Hogan MV, Chhabra AB, et al (Univ of Virginia Health System, Charlottesville; Univ of Pittsburgh School of Medicine, PA)

J Bone Joint Surg Am 95:2144-2151, 2013

Nerve injuries result in approximately $150 billion spent in annual health-care dollars in the United States. Most patients are young males, with the radial nerve in the upper extremity and the peroneal nerve in the lower extremity most commonly injured. Selecting the proper treatment continues to pose a challenging problem with a wide variability in approach and outcome. Direct tensionless end-to-end repair, when possible, achieves the most predictable outcomes. In nerve injuries when the nerve ends cannot be approximated without tension, nerve grafts represent the most commonly used method of reconstruction. The development of nerve conduits to enhance nerve repair remains an important research area and future clinical developments in the area of nerve regeneration and repair potentially could improve patient outcomes.

▶ Nerve injuries result in approximately $150 billion spent in annual health care dollars in the United States. This is a Current Concepts Review. This review is complete and gives an excellent overview of all aspects of nerve repair. This review is not for someone looking for in-depth information.

D. J. Smith, Jr, MD

Digit Replantation: Experience of Two U.S. Academic Level-I Trauma Centers

Fufa D, Calfee R, Wall L, et al (Washington Univ School of Medicine, St Louis, MO)

J Bone Joint Surg Am 95:2127-2134, 2013

Background.—Despite advances in microsurgery, digit replantation now is performed less frequently in the U.S. compared with fifteen years ago. There has been uncertainty regarding whether previously reported U.S. replantation success rates and results reported from other countries reflect the current experience in the U.S. We hypothesized that the success of digit replantation at two academic level-I referral hospitals in the U.S. would be similar to previously published results.

Methods.—In this retrospective case series, we examined all cases of digit replantation that were performed from 1997 through 2010 at two institutions. The cumulative rate of viable digit replantations was determined. Binary logistic regression modeling determined the relative impact of patient, injury, and operative factors on replantation survival.

Results.—During the study period, 135 digit replantations were performed in 106 patients. Fourteen cases did not meet our inclusion criteria, yielding a cohort of 121 replantations. The thumb (n = 40) was the most commonly replanted digit, followed by the long finger (n = 31). The mechanism of injury was classified as sharp in eighty-three digits, crush in nineteen digits, and avulsion in eighteen digits. The majority of replantations were performed following Tamai level-III (n = 49) or level-IV (n = 56) amputations. Sixty-nine (57%) of the digit, replantation procedures were successful. Logistic regression analysis identified replantation of the radial three digits and no history of tobacco use as significant independent predictors of replantation success.

Conclusions.—The rate of success of digit replantation (57%) at two academic level-I trauma hospitals was lower than previously published rates. Radial-digit involvement and no prior tobacco use were associated with replantation success. This modest success rate reflects a need for additional evaluation of our current benchmarks and clinical settings for replantation surgery. These data help to better inform patients, families, and physicians who are considering digit replantation.

▶ The rate of digital replantation has gradually decreased over the last 15 years. Two Level-I trauma centers analyzed their data during that period. They found a success rate of 57%, which is lower than previously published rates. They propose that the modest success rate causes us to reevaluate our current benchmarks and clinical settings for replantation surgery. This should also be used for patient and family counseling. This is an excellent, tight, well-done study. This report is a must for anyone doing this surgery and highly suggested to all. This should force all replantation centers to review their own experiences.

D. J. Smith, Jr, MD

Economic Analysis of Revision Amputation and Replantation Treatment of Finger Amputation Injuries

Sears ED, Shin R, Prosser LA, et al (Univ of Michigan Health System, Ann Arbor; Veterans Administration Health System, Ann Arbor, MI)

Plast Reconstr Surg 133:827-840, 2014

Background.—The purpose of this study was to perform a cost-utility analysis to compare revision amputation and replantation treatment of finger amputation injuries across a spectrum of injury scenarios.

Methods.—The study was conducted from the societal perspective. Decision tree models were created for the reference case (two-finger amputation injury) and seven additional injury scenarios for comparison. Inputs included cost, quality of life, and probability of each health state. A Web-based time trade-off survey was created to determine quality-adjusted life-years for health states; 685 nationally representative adult community members were invited to participate in the survey. Overall cost and quality-adjusted life-years for revision amputation and replantation were calculated for each decision tree. An incremental cost-effectiveness ratio was calculated if a treatment was more costly but more effective.

Results.—The authors had a 64 percent response rate ($n = 437$). Replantation treatment had greater costs and quality-adjusted life-years compared with revision amputation in all injury scenarios. Replantation of single-digit injuries had the highest incremental cost-effectiveness ratio ($136,400 per quality-adjusted life-year gained). Replantation of three- and four-digit amputation injuries had relatively low cost-to-benefit ratios ($27,100 and $23,800 per quality-adjusted life-year, respectively). Replantation for distal thumb amputation had a relatively low incremental cost-effectiveness ratio ($26,300 per quality-adjusted life-year) compared with replantation of nonthumb distal amputations ($60,200 per quality-adjusted life-year).

Conclusions.—The relative cost per quality-adjusted life-year gained with replantation treatment varied greatly among the injury scenarios. Situations in which indications for replantation are debated had higher cost per quality-adjusted life-year gained. This study highlights variability in value for replantation among different injury scenarios.

▶ This study compares the cost and quality of life associated with revision amputation and replantation treatments for multiple finger amputation injury scenarios. Replantation was more costly but more effective in all scenarios examined. Measurements of cost and quality of life associated with competing interventions will help guide policy and discussions among individual patients and physicians. Advocates of cost-effectiveness analysis argue that data should be used to identify and direct resources toward interventions having the greatest value in health care. If you're not familiar with this methodology, a must read. If you are familiar, the results are variable.

D. J. Smith, Jr, MD

Ciprofloxacin-Resistant *Aeromonas* Infection Following Leech Therapy for Digit Replantation: Report of 2 Cases

van Alphen NA, Gonzalez A, McKenna MC, et al (Mayo Clinic, Rochester, MN)

J Hand Surg Am 39:499-502, 2014

Medicinal leeches are commonly used after finger replantation to treat surgically unsalvageable venous congestion. Infection from *Aeromonas hydrophila* is a recognized complication of leech therapy that can be underestimated by the medical community. Ciprofloxacin and trimethoprim-sulfamethoxazole are the most commonly recommended prophylactic antibiotics used to prevent A. *hydrophila* infections during leech therapy. Here, we report 2 cases of ciprofloxacin-resistant *Aeromonas* infections, occurring within 4 months of each other. Both cases developed after leech therapy for unsuccessful digital replantation. These infections were successfully treated with ceftriaxone. Ciprofloxacin-resistant *Aeromonas* should be recognized when determining prophylactic antibiotic protocols for replant centers when leech therapy is used for finger replantation.

▶ The authors report 2 cases of ciprofloxacin-resistant *Aeromonas hydrophila* after leech therapy. I was unaware of this. These cases are worth noting if infection from leech therapy does not respond as expected.

D. J. Smith, Jr, MD

Evidence-Based Medicine: Carpal Tunnel Syndrome

Lalonde DH (Dalhousie Univ, Saint John, New Brunswick, Canada)

Plast Reconstr Surg 133:1234-1240, 2014

Learning Objectives.—After studying this article, the participant should be able to: 1. Describe and apply the best current high-level evidence in carpal tunnel syndrome. 2. Design a treatment plan to offer tourniquet-free, sedation-free local anesthesia for patients who wish it or who are at high risk with sedation. 3. Describe the evidence and outcomes as they relate to splinting carpal tunnel patients after surgery.

Summary.—This is the third Maintenance of Certification article on carpal tunnel syndrome. Hentz and Lalonde summarized the best literature in 2008 in the first article. The second article, by Shores and Lee, presented the best evidence regarding assessment, surgical treatment, and outcomes from the literature published between 1999 and 2009. In this article, the author has concentrated on topics not covered in depth in the first two articles and provides an update of the highest level evidence on important topics from 2009 to 2013. Although there is some Level IV and V evidence cited in this article, most is Level I, II, and III.

▶ All of the Maintenance of Certification—continuing medical education articles have been excellent. These 4 (Evidence-Based Medicine: Dupuytren Contracture, Evidence-Based Medicine: Flexor Tendon Repair, Evidence-Based Medicine: Metacarpal Fractures, Evidence-Based Medicine: Carpal Tunnel Syndrome) are no exception. The goal of the metacarpal fracture article, the flexor tendon article, and the Dupuytren contracture article is to highlight the most recent literature and the best evidence available for the management of these 3 diseases. In the carpal tunnel syndrome article, Dr Lalonde concentrates on topics not covered in depth in the first 2 articles (first article 2008, summarization of best literature; second article, best evidence for assessment, surgical treatment, and outcomes from the literature published between 1999 and 2009) and provides an update of the highest level evidence on important topics between 2009 to 2013. All 4 articles achieve their goals admirably. Must read.

D. J. Smith, Jr, MD

Carpal Tunnel Release in Patients With Diabetes: A 5-year Follow-Up With Matched Controls

Thomsen NOB, Cederlund RI, Andersson GS, et al (Lund Univ, Sweden; Skåne Univ Hosp, Lund, Sweden)

J Hand Surg Am 39:713-720, 2014

Purpose.—To compare clinical outcomes 5 years after carpal tunnel release among patients with and without diabetes.

Methods.—In a prospective consecutive series, 35 patients with diabetes (median age, 54 y; 15 type 1 and 20 type 2 diabetes) with carpal tunnel syndrome were age- and sex-matched with 31 control patients without diabetes (median age, 51 y) with idiopathic carpal tunnel syndrome. Exclusion criteria were other nerve entrapment, cervical radiculopathy, inflammatory joint disease, thyroid disorder, previous wrist fracture, and long-term exposure to vibrating tools. Participants were examined independently at baseline, 1 year, and 5 years after surgery for sensory function (Semmes-Weinstein), motor function (abductor pollicis brevis muscle strength and grip strength), cold intolerance, and completion of the Boston Carpal Tunnel Questionnaire symptom severity and functional status score.

Results.—Five years after surgery, the overall attendance rate for clinical examinations and completion of the Boston Carpal Tunnel Questionnaire were 86% and 95%, respectively. Between 1 and 5 years after surgery, there was a tendency toward a decrease in sensory function but an increase in motor function, with no statistically significant difference between groups. Cold intolerance demonstrated long-term significant improvement for patients with diabetes. The improvement in symptom severity and functional status score, as well as the large effect size, were maintained at 5 years in both patient groups.

Conclusions.—Long-term improvement in patients with diabetes remained after carpal tunnel release to the same extent as for patients without diabetes. Furthermore, improvement in cold intolerance in patients with diabetes suggests the potential for the long-term regeneration of small nerve fibers.

Type of Study/Level of Evidence.—Prognostic I.

▶ This group previously published short-term results from a prospective study on carpal tunnel release among age- and sex-matched patients with and without diabetes. This investigation was to extend their clinical trial to compare outcomes 5 years after open carpal tunnel release in patients with and without diabetes. They found long-term improvement in patients after carpal tunnel release to the same extent as for patients without diabetes. There was also improvement in cold intolerance in the diabetes group. This is a very well done study. By publishing the original results and now following up with 5-year results, the authors certainly provide support for operative treatment of patients with carpal tunnel syndrome.

D. J. Smith, Jr, MD

Evidence-Based Medicine: Dupuytren Contracture

Eaton C (The Hand Ctr, Jupiter, FL)

Plast Reconstr Surg 133:1241-1251, 2014

Learning Objectives.—After studying this article, the participant should be able to: 1. Describe features and clinical importance of Dupuytren diathesis. 2. Explain the difference between the new definition of recurrence used in collagenase studies compared with prior definitions of recurrence. 3. Compare and list the main advantage/main disadvantage of fasciectomy versus minimally invasive treatment (collagenase injection or needle aponeurotomy) of Dupuytren contracture.

Summary.—The large body of existing literature on Dupuytren disease is spread across many journals in many specialties. It is thus a daunting task for practitioners to follow trends and practice recommendations. It is also a testimony to the lack of an acceptable solution to this common problem. Recent publications provide evidence to highlight controversies and challenge some traditional teachings. Literature from 2010 to 2012 was reviewed with the intent of clarifying some of these issues.

▶ All of the Maintenance of Certification—continuing medical education articles have been excellent. These 4 (Evidence-Based Medicine: Dupuytren Contracture, Evidence-Based Medicine: Flexor Tendon Repair, Evidence-Based Medicine: Metacarpal Fractures, Evidence-Based Medicine: Carpal Tunnel Syndrome) are no exception. The goal of the metacarpal fracture article, the flexor tendon article, and the Dupuytren contracture article is to highlight the most recent literature and the best evidence available for the management of these 3 diseases. In the carpal tunnel syndrome article, Dr Lalonde concentrates on topics not covered in depth in the first 2 articles (first article 2008, summarization of best literature; second article, best evidence for assessment, surgical treatment, and outcomes from the literature published between 1999 and 2009) and provides an update of the highest level evidence on important topics between 2009 to 2013. All 4 articles achieve their goals admirably. Must read.

D. J. Smith, Jr, MD

Dupuytren Disease: European Hand Surgeons, Hand Therapists, and Physical Medicine and Rehabilitation Physicians Agree on a Multidisciplinary Treatment Guideline: Results from the HANDGUIDE Study

Huisstede BMA, On behalf of the European HANDGUIDE Group (Erasmus MC-Univ Med Ctr Rotterdam, the Netherlands; et al)

Plast Reconstr Surg 132:964e-976e, 2013

Background.—Multidisciplinary treatment guidelines for Dupuytren disease can aid in optimizing the quality of care for patients with this disorder. Therefore, this study aimed to achieve consensus on a multidisciplinary treatment guideline for Dupuytren disease.

Methods.—A European Delphi consensus strategy was initiated. A systematic review reporting on the effectiveness of interventions was conducted and used as an evidence-based starting point for this study. In total, 39 experts (hand surgeons, hand therapists, and physical medicine and rehabilitation physicians) participated in the Delphi consensus strategy. Each Delphi round consisted of a questionnaire, an analysis, and a feedback report.

Results.—After four Delphi rounds, consensus was achieved on the description, symptoms, and diagnosis of Dupuytren disease. No nonsurgical interventions were included in the guideline. Needle and open fasciotomy, and a limited fasciectomy and dermofasciectomy, were seen as suitable surgical techniques for Dupuytren disease. Factors relevant for choosing one of these surgical techniques were identified and divided into patient-related (age, comorbidity), disease-related (palpable cord, previous surgery in the same area, skin involvement, time of recovery, recurrences), and surgeon-related (years of experience) factors. Associations of these factors with the choice of a specific surgical technique were reported in the guideline. Postsurgical rehabilitation should always include instructions and exercise therapy; postsurgical splinting should be performed on indication. Relevant details for the use of surgical and postsurgical interventions were described.

Conclusion.—This treatment guideline is likely to promote further discussion on related clinical and scientific issues and may therefore contribute to better treatment of patients with Dupuytren disease.

▶ The authors achieved a consensus on a multidisciplinary treatment guideline for Dupuytren disease. The process and completeness are absolutely amazing. This is the first time that a multidisciplinary treatment guideline was developed in cooperation with experts from all over Europe. I assume we will be seeing more attempts to gain this type of consensus. For that reason, this is a highly recommended read into the future.

D. J. Smith, Jr, MD

Health-Related Quality of Life in Patients Undergoing Palmar Fasciectomy for Dupuytren's Disease

Thoma A, Kaur MN, Ignacy TA, et al (McMaster Univ, Hamilton, Toronto, Canada; Univ of Toronto, Ontario, Canada)

Plast Reconstr Surg 133:1411-1419, 2014

Background.—The present study was undertaken to assess the health-related quality of life in patients with Dupuytren's disease who undergo palmar fasciectomy.

Methods.—A prospective cohort of patients with Dupuytren's disease undergoing palmar and/or digital fasciectomy was recruited from the practice of three plastic surgeons in Hamilton, Ontario, Canada. After written informed consent was obtained, participants were asked to complete three health-related quality-of-life questionnaires (i.e., Short Form-36, Michigan Hand Outcomes Questionnaire, and Health Utility Index Mark 3) at five time points: at 1 week and 1 day preoperatively, and at 1, 3, 6, and 12 months postoperatively. Ranges of motion and grip strength measurement were also recorded.

Results.—For the 26 patients in the study, the multiattribute scores of the Health Utility Index Mark 3 improved from 0.80 before surgery to 0.83 at 12 months postoperatively ($p > 0.05$). There was no difference in the Short Form-36 scores, but the Michigan Hand Outcomes Questionnaire scores improved from 74 at 1 week preoperatively to 90 at the 12-month postoperative visit ($p < 0.001$).

Conclusions.—Patients who undergo palmar fasciectomy for Dupuytren's disease experience a substantial improvement in their health-related quality of life 12 months after surgery. In the authors' study population, a benefit of 0.85 quality-adjusted life-year within 12 months was observed. This can be translated as follows: the average patient who undergoes palmar fasciectomy gains the equivalent of approximately 14.4 days (0.48 months) in perfect health by undergoing palmar fasciectomy.

Clinical Question/Level of Evidence.—Therapeutic, I

▶ This study was done to assess health-related quality of life in patients with Dupuytren disease who undergo palmar fasciectomy. This is the first study to prospectively measure the utilities in patients undergoing surgical management for Dupuytren disease using patient-based data. The study adds significantly to the limited evidence that exists for the use of self-reported outcomes in Dupuytren disease and provides the platform on which future randomized studies can be based. Furthermore, the effect size identified in this study can be used as the minimal clinical important difference to calculate the sample size in future randomized trials. An excellent study in its own right, it is more important to understand because of the outcomes parameters and how they were used.

D. J. Smith, Jr, MD

Efficacy and Safety of Concurrent Collagenase Clostridium Histolyticum Injections for Multiple Dupuytren Contractures

Coleman S, Gilpin D, Kaplan FTD, et al (Brisbane Hand and Upper Limb Clinic, Queensland, Australia; Indiana Hand to Shoulder Ctr, Indianapolis; Caboolture Clinical Res Centre, Queensland, Australia; et al)

J Hand Surg Am 39:57-64, 2014

Purpose.—To assess the safety and efficacy of 2 concurrent injections of collagenase clostridium histolyticum (CCH) in the same hand to treat multiple Dupuytren flexion contractures.

Methods.—In a multicenter, open-label phase IIIb study, 60 patients received two 0.58-mg CCH doses injected into cords affecting 2 joints in the same hand during 1 visit, followed by finger extension approximately 24 hours later. Efficacy at postinjection day 30 (change in flexion contracture and active range of motion, patient satisfaction, physician-rated improvement, and rates of clinical success [flexion contracture 5° or less]) and adverse events were summarized.

Results.—The concurrent injections were most commonly administered in cords affecting metacarpophalangeal (MCP) and proximal interphalangeal (PIP) joints on the same finger (47%) or 2 MCP joints on different fingers of the same hand (37%). Mean total (sum of the 2 treated joints) flexion contracture decreased 76%, from 87° to 24° (MCP joints: 86%; PIP joints: 66%). Mean total range of motion increased from 100° to 161°. Clinical success was 76% for MCP joints and 33% for PIP joints. Most patients were very satisfied (60%) or quite satisfied (28%) with treatment. Most investigators rated treated joints as very much improved (55%) or much improved (37%). The most common treatment-related adverse events (>75% of patients) were contusion, pain in extremity, and edema peripheral (local edema). Most adverse events were mild to moderate in severity. Serious complications included 1 pulley rupture related to study medication and 1 flexor tendon rupture (following conclusion of the study). There were no systemic complications.

Conclusions.—Results suggest that 2 affected joints can be effectively and safely treated with concurrent CCH injections. There was an increased incidence of some adverse events with concurrent treatment (pruritus, lymphadenopathy, blood blister, and skin laceration) compared with treatment of a single joint. High degrees of patient satisfaction and physician-rated improvement were reported.

Type of Study/Level of Evidence.—Therapeutic IV.

▶ The authors report that 2 affected joints can be effectively and safely treated with concurrent collagenase clostridium histolyticum injections in Dupuytren's contracture. There was an increased incidence of some adverse events with concurrent treatment (pruritus, lymphadenopathy, blood blister, and skin laceration). High degrees of patient satisfaction and physician-rated improvement are reported. This treatment modality is clearly here to stay. We will see more studies looking at expanding or altering types, number, area of injection. As an aside, residents are increasingly having difficulty meeting the minimum number of open procedures on their operative logs. It makes one wonder if we are training a generation of hand surgeons who won't feel comfortable with the open procedure.

D. J. Smith, Jr, MD

Technical Tips for Collagenase Injection Treatment for Dupuytren Contracture

Meals RA, Hentz VR (Univ of California at Los Angeles; Stanford Univ, CA)
J Hand Surg Am 39:1195-1200.e2, 2014

We describe technical tips for injecting collagenase into Dupuytren cords based on experience acquired during the prerelease Food and Drug Administration clinical trials and with subsequent clinical practice. These tips include techniques for extracting the reconstituted enzyme efficiently from the vial, injecting the cord(s) with increased safety to the tendons, and anesthetizing the hand before manipulation. The tips are intended to supplement but by no means replace the manufacturer's prescribing information and training video.

▶ The authors describe technical tips for injecting collagenase into Dupuytren cords based on experience acquired during the prerelease Food and Drug Administration clinical trials and with subsequent clinical practice. The tips discuss injection techniques, manipulation techniques, postinjection management, and complications. Why not learn from this extensive experience? A must for anyone using this technique.

D. J. Smith, Jr, MD

Free Function Muscle Transfers for Upper Extremity Reconstruction: A Review of Indications, Techniques, and Outcomes

Fischer JP, Elliott RM, Kozin SH, et al (Hosp of the Univ of Pennsylvania, Philadelphia; Shriners Hosp for Children, Philadelphia, PA)
J Hand Surg Am 38:2485-2490, 2013

Free functional muscle transfer (FFMT) replaces destroyed, denervated, or resected skeletal muscle units in the upper extremity with functioning skeletal muscle from other locations in the body. Common indications for FFMT include brachial plexus injuries, ischemic contracture, tumor resection, and extensive direct muscle trauma. Recent studies have focused on improving patient outcomes through refinements in muscle flap harvest and inset, donor nerve selection, and postoperative management. In this review, we assess and summarize the current literature on FFMT, with emphasis on etiopathogenesis, diagnosis, treatment, postoperative management, and clinical outcomes.

▶ The authors review free functional muscle transfers (FFMT). They evaluate the current literature on FFMT, with emphasis on etiopathogenesis, diagnosis, treatment, postoperative management, and clinical outcomes. This is an excellent read for all, regardless of whether you are doing microsurgery.

D. J. Smith, Jr, MD

The safety and efficacy of epinephrine in hand surgery: a systematic review of the literature and international survey

Shridharani SM, Manson PN, Magarakis M, et al (Manhattan Eye, Ear, and Throat Hosp, NY; The Johns Hopkins Univ School of Medicine, Baltimore, MD; Univ of Maryland School of Medicine, Baltimore; et al)

Eur J Plast Surg 37:183-188, 2014

The concept that epinephrine-based local anesthetics cannot be injected in terminal appendages has been perpetuated for decades. The hypothesis that the vasoconstrictive effect of epinephrine will result in finger necrosis has been accepted as fact, often preventing its use in hand surgery. To scientifically challenge this hypothesis, a systematic review of the literature was performed, and a survey of ASPS members reported to highlight the lack of evidence-based opinions. A systematic literature review performed using Medline, Embase, PubMed, and Cochrane databases identified all published studies evaluating use of epinephrine/adrenaline in hand, finger or digit surgery. Each study was independently evaluated by three reviewers for inclusion or exclusion from the systematic review. Additionally, a survey (E-survey link) was distributed to all ASPS members and data were collected over a 5-month period through SurveyMonkey®. A total of 568 articles published prior to December 2012 were identified. After elimination of 151 duplicates, 417 articles remained. Fifty-five articles were selected and full examination of the texts was performed. Forty-five studies matched the selection criteria and were included in the analysis. The ASPS member survey demonstrated a 13 % overall questionnaire response rate (5,299 questionnaires/687 responses). Of all respondents, 37.4 % felt it was unsafe to inject local anesthesia mixed with epinephrine into the fingers/thumb, respectively. Critical literature review validated the safety and efficacy of utilizing epinephrine-based local anesthetics. The author's survey elucidates the pervasive concern of employing epinephrine in hand surgery.

► The concept that epinephrine-based local anesthesia cannot be injected in terminal appendages has been perpetuated for decades. Recently, Dr Don Lalonde and others have challenged this concept with their hand surgery using local anesthesia. These authors have done a complete review of the literature and conclude that it is safe and effective to use epinephrine-based local anesthetics in terminal appendages. This is an exhaustive, comprehensive review of the literature and a must for anyone remotely considering using epinephrine-based local anesthetics in these situations.

D. J. Smith, Jr, MD

Dosage of Local Anesthesia in Wide Awake Hand Surgery

Lalonde DH, Wong A (Dalhousie Univ, Saint John, New Brunswick, Canada; Dalhousie Univ, Halifax, Nova Scotia, Canada)
J Hand Surg 38A:2025-2028, 2013

Background.—Patients having wide awake hand surgery express satisfaction with the process because it requires no preoperative testing, causes no tourniquet pain, shortens surgery, allows them to communicate during surgery, and does not produce cloudy thinking postoperatively. The principles and procedures of tumescent local anesthesia were discussed.

Principles.—Lidocaine with epinephrine is injected subcutaneously only where needed, which is where the surgeon will dissect, move fractures, or insert K-wires. Tourniquets are replaced by epinephrine for hemostasis, and a smaller (25-gauge) needle is used at a slower pace of injection.

Lidocaine is preferred over bupivacaine to avoid the cardiotoxicity and morbidity of intravascular bupivacaine as well as the annoying touch and pressure numbness that follow its short pain-relieving effect. In addition, the lidocaine-epinephrine combination has proved safe in dentistry for over 60 years. When a procedure is likely to last longer than 2.5 hours, 10 ml of 0.5% bupivacaine with 1:200,000 epinephrine can be added to the total injectate so the patient does not experience a decline in pain amelioration.

Injections are done while the patient is on a stretcher outside the operating room. This allows more time for the epinephrine to reach the maximal optimal vasoconstriction time of 26 minutes, avoids the vasovagal reaction leading to fainting that occurs when patients sit up during injection, and does not waste valuable operating time.

Procedures.—Injection begins slowly with 2 ml of lidocaine with epinephrine just below the skin. Small subcutaneous veins are avoided by collapsing them using antegrade injection. At least 1 cm of visible or palpable local anesthesia ahead of the sharp needle tip is required to avoid pain. Large areas are anesthetized by reinserting the needle within 1 cm of visible palpable local anesthesia. Slow injection pace diminishes pain. Patients can be asked to report the number of times they feel pain during injection. By the end of the injection, the patient should have at least 1 cm of adrenalized skin beyond all borders of incision and dissection sites.

The accepted maximal lidocaine plus epinephrine dosage is 7 mg/kg, meaning an average 70-kg person can safely receive 50 ml of 1% lidocaine with epinephrine. If a smaller dose is needed, 1% lidocaine with 1:100,000 epinephrine can be used. If a larger dose is needed, ½% lidocaine with 1:200,000 epinephrine provides a 50 to 100 ml volume, and ¼% lidocaine with 1:400,000 epinephrine provides a 100 to 200 ml volume. The preferred ratio to neutralize the acidic pH of 1% lidocaine with 1:100,000 epinephrine is 10 ml lidocaine to 1 ml 8.4% bicarbonate, which minimizes injection pain.

Between 50 and 100 ml of 0.5% lidocaine with 1:200,000 epinephrine is injected from proximal to distal when dissection is required for spaghetti wrist and ulnar nerve decompression at the elbow. Forearm transfers require up to 200 ml ¼% lidocaine with 1:400,000 epinephrine, with bupivacaine added to extend coverage. Sensory nerves must be bathed in local anesthesia for wrist or forearm procedures, but forearm motor nerves should remain intact to test active movement of the repaired or transferred structures.

Conclusions.—Tumescent local anesthesia places lidocaine and epinephrine where needed and avoids complications while enhancing patient convenience.

▶ Dr Lalonde has long championed local anesthesia in wide-awake hand surgery. He notes that patients benefit from (1) no preoperative testing, (2) no tourniquet pain, (3) less time at the hospital to have surgery, (4) the ability to speak to their surgeon during the surgery, and (5) no sedation to cloud their head when they get home from their surgery. This article is a "how to" article. It addresses technique, dosage, choice of agent, and large-volume injection. This is an excellent article only for those interested in the technique.

D. J. Smith, Jr, MD

Treatment of Complex Soft-Tissue Defects at the Metacarpophalangeal Joint of the Thumb Using the Bilobed Second Dorsal Metacarpal Artery–Based Island Flap

Zhu H, Zhang X, Yan M, et al (The Second Hosp of Qinhuangdao, Changli, Hebei, People's Republic of China)

Plast Reconstr Surg 131:1091-1097, 2013

Background.—The purpose of this study is to report on reconstruction of complex soft-tissue defects around the metacarpophalangeal joint of the thumb using a bilobed second dorsal metacarpal artery–based island flap taken from the dorsum of the proximal phalanges of the index and long fingers.

Methods.—From March of 2007 to October of 2009, the bilobed second dorsal metacarpal artery–based island flap was transferred in 13 patients. There were two defects on the metacarpophalangeal joint of the thumb. The mean size of the dorsal defects was 2.4 × 3.2 cm; the mean size of the volar defects was 2.6 × 4.0 cm. The mean size of the flaps taken from the index and long fingers was 2.6 × 3.4 cm and 2.8 × 3.2 cm, respectively. The mean pedicle length was 4.9 cm.

Results.—All flaps survived completely. At a mean follow-up of 14 months, the mean active motion arc of the thumb metacarpophalangeal joints was 42 degrees. The motion of the donor fingers was similar to that on the opposite side. The mean values of static two-point discrimination of the donor sites of the index and long fingers were 6 and 7 mm, respectively.

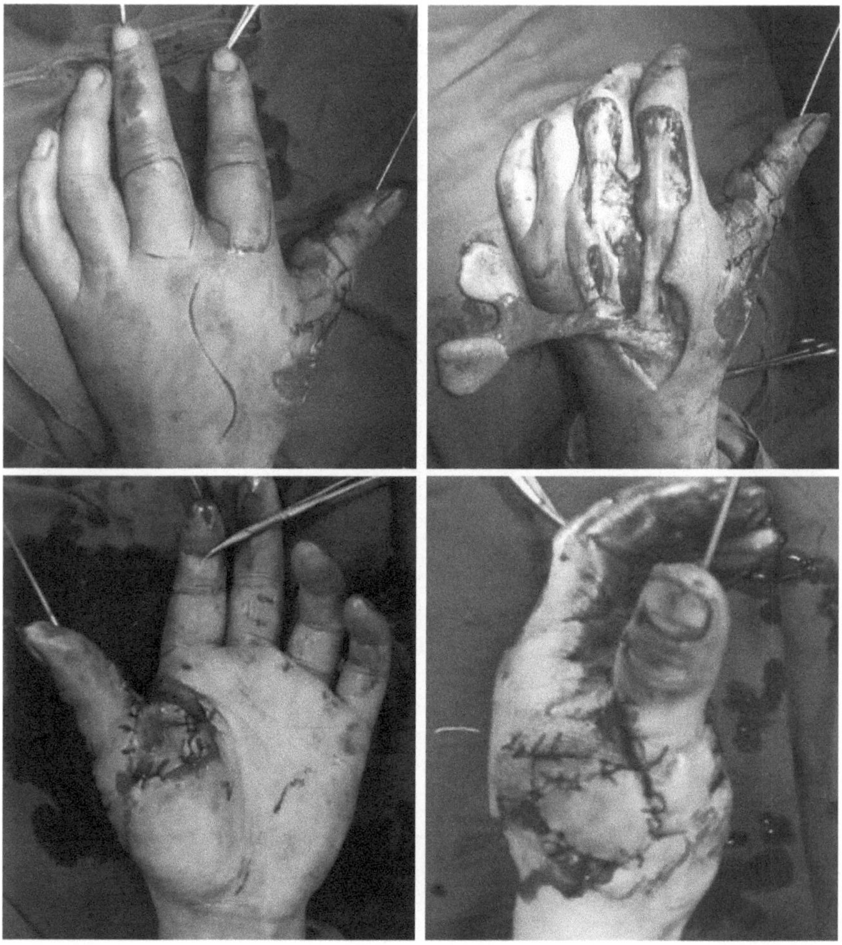

FIGURE 3.—(*Above, left*) Flap design. (*Above, right*) Flap harvesting is complete. (*Below, left*) Volar defect is covered with the flap taken from the long finger. (*Below, right*) Dorsal defect is covered with the flap taken from the index finger. (Reprinted from Zhu H, Zhang X, Yan M, et al. Treatment of complex soft-tissue defects at the metacarpophalangeal joint of the thumb using the bilobed second dorsal metacarpal artery–based island flap. *Plast Reconstr Surg*. 2013;131:1091-1097, with permission from the American Society of Plastic Surgeons.)

Conclusion.—Transferring the bilobed second dorsal metacarpal artery–based island flap is a useful and reliable technique for reconstructing complex defects around the metacarpophalangeal joint of the thumb.

Clinical Question/Level of Evidence.—Therapeutic IV (Figs 3 and 4).

▶ This study is a particularly worthwhile addition to the armamentarium of hand surgeons dealing with complex soft tissue injuries involving the metacarpophalangeal joint of the thumb. Modification of the flap to exclude the first

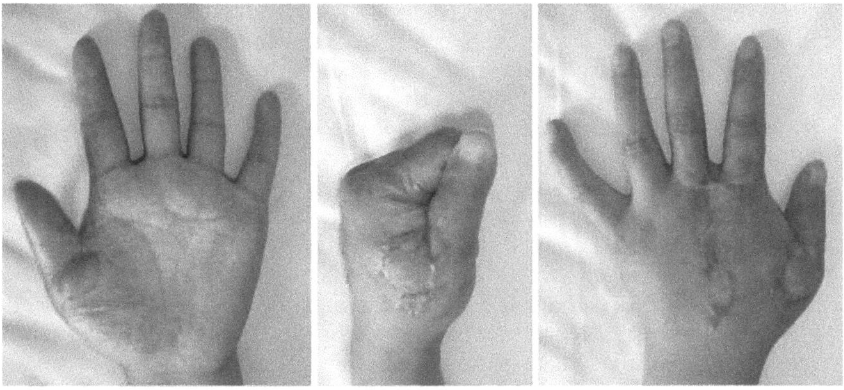

FIGURE 4.—Results after 13 months. (*Left*) Extension. (*Center*) Flexion. (*Right*) Donor sites. (Reprinted from Zhu H, Zhang X, Yan M, et al. Treatment of complex soft-tissue defects at the metacarpophalangeal joint of the thumb using the bilobed second dorsal metacarpal artery—based island flap. *Plast Reconstr Surg*. 2013;131:1091-1097, with permission from the American Society of Plastic Surgeons.)

dorsal metacarpal artery but to include the second metacarpal artery to create a bilobed island flap of skin from the index and long fingers allows harvesting of enough tissue to allow coverage of a sizable volar and dorsal defect. The major difficulty seems to be tethering of the web space between the thumb and the index finger. Other problems, such as tendon adherence and decreased joint, are also reported and said to be caused by the primary injury rather than the use of the flap.

S. H. Miller, MD

Nerve

Functional Outcome Thirty Years After Median and Ulnar Nerve Repair in Childhood and Adolescence

Chemnitz A, Björkman A, Dahlin LB, et al (Skåne Univ Hosp, Malmö, Sweden)
J Bone Joint Surg Am 95:329-337, 2013

Background.—Age at injury is believed to be a factor that strongly influences functional outcome after nerve injury. However, there have been few long-term evaluations of the results of nerve repair and reconstruction in children. Our aim was to evaluate the long-term functional outcome of nerve repair or reconstruction at the forearm level in patients with a complete median and/or ulnar nerve injury at a young age.

Methods.—Forty-five patients were assessed at a median of thirty-one years after a complete median and/or ulnar nerve injury in the forearm. The outcome was classified with a total score (the Rosén score), a standardized outcome instrument consisting of three separate domains for sensory and motor function as well as pain/discomfort. In addition, the DASH (Disabilities of the Arm, Shoulder and Hand) score, sensitivity to cold, and locognosia were assessed specifically, together with the patient's estimation of the overall outcome and impact on his or her education, work, and leisure activities. Comparisons were made between injuries that occurred in childhood (less than twelve years of age) and those that were sustained in adolescence (twelve to twenty years of age), and according to the nerve(s) that was injured (median nerve, ulnar nerve, or both).

Results.—Functional recovery, expressed as the total outcome score, the sensory domain of that score, and the patient's subjective estimation of outcome, was significantly better after injuries sustained in childhood than after those that occurred in adolescence (87% and 67% of complete recovery, respectively; $p < 0.001$). No significant differences in recovery were seen between median and ulnar nerve injuries, or even when both nerves were injured. Motor function was close to normal, and cold sensitivity was not a problem in either age group. The median DASH scores were within normal limits and did not differ between the groups. Patients who sustained the injury in adolescence indicated that the nerve injury had a significantly higher effect on their profession, education, and leisure activities.

Conclusions.—At a median of thirty-one years after a median or ulnar nerve repair at the level of the forearm, nerve function is significantly better in those injured in childhood than in those injured in adolescence, with almost full sensory and motor recovery in individuals injured in childhood.

▶ Functional wisdom has taught that the younger the patient, the better the anticipated outcome after injury. These authors evaluated the long-term functional outcome of nerve repair or reconstruction at the forearm level in patients with a complete median or ulnar nerve injury at a young age. At a median of 31 years after a medial or ulnar nerve repair at the level of the forearm, nerve function was significantly better in those injured in childhood than in those injured in adolescence, with almost full sensory recovery in individuals injured in childhood. Patients who sustained the injury in adolescence indicated that the nerve injury had a significantly higher effect on their profession, education, and leisure activities.

This is a well-done study and the length of follow-up is impressive. Unfortunately, there were several missing patients, which may raise the question of selection bias. However, the length of follow-up trumps that possibility.

D. J. Smith, Jr, MD

5 Aesthetic

General and Anesthesia

A Comparative Analysis of Readmission Rates After Outpatient Cosmetic Surgery

Mioton LM, Alghoul MS, Kim JYS (Vanderbilt Univ School of Medicine, Nashville, TN; Northwestern Univ, Chicago, IL)

Aesthet Surg J 34:317-323, 2014

Background.—Despite the increasing scrutiny of surgical procedures, outpatient cosmetic surgery has an established record of safety and efficacy. A key measure in assessing surgical outcomes is the examination of readmission rates. However, there is a paucity of data on unplanned readmission following cosmetic surgery procedures.

Objectives.—The authors studied readmission rates for outpatient cosmetic surgery and compared the data with readmission rates for other surgical procedures.

Methods.—The 2011 National Surgical Quality Improvement Program (NSQIP) data set was queried for all outpatient procedures. Readmission rates were calculated for the 5 surgical specialties with the greatest number of outpatient procedures and for the overall outpatient cosmetic surgery population. Subgroup analysis was performed on the 5 most common cosmetic surgery procedures. Multivariate regression models were used to determine predictors of readmission for cosmetic surgery patients.

Results.—The 2879 isolated outpatient cosmetic surgery cases had an associated 0.90% unplanned readmission rate. The 5 specialties with the highest number of outpatient surgical procedures were general, orthopedic, gynecologic, urologic, and otolaryngologic surgery; their unplanned readmission rates ranged from 1.21% to 3.73%. The 5 most common outpatient cosmetic surgery procedures and their associated readmission rates were as follows: reduction mammaplasty, 1.30%; mastopexy, 0.31%; liposuction, 1.13%; abdominoplasty, 1.78%; and breast augmentation, 1.20%. Multivariate regression analysis demonstrated that operating time (in hours) was an independent predictor of readmission (odds ratio, 1.40; 95% confidence interval, 1.08-1.81; $P = .010$).

Conclusions.—Rates of unplanned readmission with outpatient cosmetic surgery are low and compare favorably to those of other outpatient surgeries.

▶ Although it appears that outpatient aesthetic surgery has a lower readmission rate than other surgical specialties, there is room for improvement. Although this report does not offer guidance on a reasonable length of surgery, it was the only variable that was associated with readmission.

K. A. Gutowski, MD

Psychological Screening Measures for Cosmetic Plastic Surgery Patients: A Systematic Review

Wildgoose P, Scott A, Pusic AL, et al (McMaster Univ, Hamilton, Ontario, Canada; Memorial Sloan-Kettering Cancer Ctr, NY; et al)

Aesthet Surg J 33:152-159, 2013

With the increasing popularity of cosmetic surgery procedures, preoperative psychological assessment of cosmetic surgery patients may improve outcomes by highlighting patient expectations and motivations, as well as by identifying those who may require psychological referral. In this article, the authors describe a systematic literature review to identify and evaluate current self-report tools used in the psychological screening of cosmetic surgery patients prior to surgery. Articles related to the preoperative mental health assessment of cosmetic surgery patients were identified by searching MEDLINE, EMBASE, HAPI, CINAHL, PsycINFO, and the Cochrane Central Register of Controlled Trials through November 2010. The full text of potentially relevant articles was examined by 2 reviewers, and articles that met the inclusion criteria were reported. Close reading of 100 full-text articles showed that although a variety of instruments are currently being used as preoperative assessment tools, there are limitations to their validity and usefulness in the screening of cosmetic surgery patients. To properly assess cosmetic surgery patients, a scientifically sound and clinically useful instrument is needed.

▶ Patients seeking cosmetic procedures seem to have a disproportionate tendency of meeting the criteria for a psychiatric disorder such as body dysmorphic disorder, narcissistic personality disorder, or histrionic personality disorder. Such patients are more likely to be dissatisfied after surgery and may have further progression of psychiatric symptoms. Unfortunately, a validated and easy-to-use screening mechanism specific for this purpose has not yet been developed. Until it is, surgeons must remain vigilant when assessing patients for procedures.

K. A. Gutowski, MD

The Measurable Cost of Complications for Outpatient Cosmetic Surgery in Patients With Mental Health Diagnoses

Wimalawansa SM, Fox JP, Johnson RM (Wright State Univ, Dayton, OH)
Aesthet Surg J 34:306-316, 2014

Background.—Mental health conditions, including psychiatric and substance abuse diagnoses, have been associated with poor postoperative outcomes, but no studies have quantified the relationship to date.

Objective.—The authors examine the association between mental health conditions and immediate postoperative outcomes as defined by further hospital-based acute care within 30 days of surgery.

Methods.—California State Ambulatory Surgery, Inpatient, and Emergency Department Databases were used to identify all adult patients undergoing outpatient cosmetic plastic surgery between January 2007 and October 2011. Patients were subgrouped by the presence of mental health or substance abuse conditions. Primary outcome was the need for hospital-based acute care (admission or emergency department visit) within 30 days after surgery. Multivariable logistic regression models compared outcomes between groups.

Results.—Of 116 597 patients meeting inclusion criteria, 3.9% and 1.4% had either a psychiatric or substance abuse diagnosis, respectively. Adjusting for medical comorbidities, patients with psychiatric disorders more frequently required hospital-based acute care within 30 days postoperatively than those without mental illness diagnoses (11.1% vs 3.6%; adjusted odds ratio [AOR], 1.78 [95% confidence interval, 1.59-1.99]). This was true both for hospital admissions (3.5% vs 1.1%; AOR, 1.61 [1.32-1.95]) and emergency department visits (8.8% vs 2.7%; AOR, 1.88 [1.66-2.14]). The most common acute diagnoses were surgical in nature, including postoperative infection, hemorrhage, and hematoma; the median hospital admission charge was $35 637. Similar findings were noted among patients with a substance abuse diagnosis.

Conclusions.—Mental health conditions are independently associated with the need for more frequent hospital-based acute care following surgery, thus contributing to added costs of care. A patients mental health should be preoperatively assessed and appropriately addressed before proceeding with any elective procedure.

Level of Evidence.—4.

► The complication rate requiring hospital or emergency department (ED) visits in cosmetic surgery patients with a mental health diagnosis is surprisingly high (3.5% and 8.8%, respectively). Many of the ED visits were because of surgical complications and pain, suggesting that better patient discussions and instructions should be provided so that patients don't have to rely on the ED to address issues that can be handled in a clinic or office setting. It may be possible that patients with a mental health diagnosis have altered perceptions of pain, nausea, and fatigue that could lead to more frequent hospital-based care after surgery and additional costs.

K. A. Gutowski, MD

Patterns of Preoperative Laboratory Testing in Patients Undergoing Outpatient Plastic Surgery Procedures

Fischer JP, Shang EK, Nelson JA, et al (Hosp of the Univ of Pennsylvania, Philadelphia)

Aesthet Surg J 34:133-141, 2014

Background.—Preoperative laboratory testing is commonplace in the clinical setting and is often utilized at surgeon discretion. We searched the American College of Surgeons–National Surgical Quality Improvement Program (ACS-NSQIP) data set to determine the impact of preoperative laboratory testing in ambulatory plastic surgery patients.

Objective.—The authors assess the utilization and predictive value of preoperative laboratory testing in outpatient plastic surgery procedures.

Methods.—Patients undergoing ambulatory plastic surgery were identified from the 2005 to 2010 NSQIP databases. Laboratory tests were categorized by group: hematologic, chemistry, coagulation, and liver function tests (LFT). We defined complications in 2 groups: major postoperative and wound complications. Multivariate analyses were used to identify patient characteristics associated with testing and to assess the ability of laboratory testing to predict postoperative complications.

Results.—A total of 5359 (62.0%) patients underwent testing; 881 (16.4%) tests were performed on the day of surgery. In patients with no defined NSQIP comorbidities, 59.4% underwent preoperative testing and had a significantly lower rate of abnormal findings (33.4% vs 25.3%, $P < .0001$). In multivariate analyses, testing was associated with older age, American Society of Anesthesiologists class >2, Hispanic or African American race, body contouring procedures, epidural or spinal procedures, and with diabetes, hypertension, and cancer. Major complications occurred in 0.34% of patients. Our analysis demonstrated that neither testing nor abnormal results were associated with postoperative complications, either major ($P = .178$) or wound ($P = .150$).

Conclusions.—We found no association between abnormal laboratory testing and postoperative morbidity. Preoperative testing in low-risk ambulatory plastic surgery patients may be costly and has limited direct clinical benefit.

▶ This article supports other studies that have questioned the use of routine preoperative laboratory blood tests before elective, low-risk surgery in asymptomatic and clinically health patients. A proper history and physical examination with evidence-based testing is more likely to be cost-effective and minimize patient inconvenience. The most recent American Society of Anesthesiologists

Practice Advisory for Preanesthesia Evaluation is available at https://www.asahq.org/For-Members/Practice-Management/Practice-Parameters.aspx.

K. A. Gutowski, MD

Corticosteroid Use in Cosmetic Plastic Surgery

Pulikkottil BJ, Dauwe P, Daniali L, et al (Univ of Texas Southwestern Med Ctr, Dallas; Rutgers New Jersey Med School, Newark)

Plast Reconstr Surg 132:352e-360e, 2013

Background.—Steroids have been used in cosmetic plastic surgery to reduce postoperative edema and ecchymosis. We performed a systematic review of the literature addressing postoperative steroid use after rhinoplasty. Due to a paucity of studies, a review of the literature was also performed for postoperative steroid use in rhytidectomy and body contouring surgery.

Methods.—An exhaustive literature search was performed using: MEDLINE, Cochrane Database of Systematic Reviews, Cochrane Central Register of Controlled Trials, and PubMed. A total of 12 articles were chosen to be included in the rhinoplasty systematic review. Cohen's kappa for level of agreement between the two reviewers was 1.0. Data recorded from each of the studies included: author, year, sample size, age, follow-up, statistical analyses, eyelid/edema assessment, significant findings, p values, and steroid regimens. A general review of the current rhytidectomy and body contouring literature associated with corticosteroids was performed as well.

Results.—No statistically significant long-term reduction in postoperative edema or ecchymosis after rhinoplasty. Significant reductions were noted in the short term (<2 days). Review of the rhytidectomy literature described no significant decrease in postoperative edema or ecchymosis. Steroid use was noted to reduce postoperative nausea and vomiting when combined with other therapies in body contouring.

Conclusions.—Steroid use is not warranted in the postoperative period and only reduces transient edema and ecchymosis. A significant benefit for steroid use after rhytidectomy is not evident as well. Steroid use may benefit in postoperative nausea and vomiting.

▶ This review is worth reading to reinforce the unfortunate fact that in an era of evidence-based medicine, many surgeons still practice without considering if their treatments are supported by science. The use of postoperative steroids for edema reduction after rhinoplasty and facial rhytidectomy does not seem to be supported by published studies and should be abandoned.

K. A. Gutowski, MD

Skin, Soft Tissue, Fillers, Hair

Applications of Fat Grafting in Facial Aesthetic Skeletal Surgery

Endara MR, Allred LJ, Han KD, et al (Georgetown Univ Hosp, Washington, DC)

Aesthet Surg J 34:363-373, 2014

Background.—Aesthetic skeletal surgery of the face is a powerful tool to alter the facial skeleton; the facial form is enhanced through the use of alloplastic implants and osteotomies of the facial bones. However, the ultimate aesthetic appearance is dictated by how the soft tissue envelope drapes over the altered skeletal foundation. Intraoperative and postoperative fat grafting enhances the final aesthetic result in patients who undergo skeletal aesthetic procedures.

Objectives.—The authors describe cases in which selective fat grafting has been successful in optimizing facial soft tissue symmetry in patients undergoing skeletal aesthetic surgery of the face.

Methods.—A retrospective chart review of all patients who underwent aesthetic skeletal surgery of the face between November 1, 2003, and October 31, 2011, in the Department of Surgery at Georgetown University Hospital was performed, and any patient who required fat grafting either at the time of aesthetic facial skeletal surgery or in the postoperative period was identified (n = 21). Common indications for fat grafting and the surgical plans are reviewed and presented in this article.

Results.—Twenty-one patients were identified who required 37 fat grafting procedures either at the time of aesthetic skeletal surgery of the face or in the postoperative period. The procedures most frequently requiring fat grafting were genioplasty, facial shape modifications, and facial symmetry improvement. Fat grafting most commonly corrected irregularities or asymmetries and improved the soft tissue contour overlying repositioned bone or alloplastic implants. Most patients were female (72%) with a mean age of 42 years (range, 4-58 years). There were 4 complications in total: 3 surgical site infections (managed conservatively in 1 patient and with incision and drainage in the remaining 2) and 1 hematoma requiring drainage and closure on the day of surgery.

Conclusions.—Knowledge of which procedures are likely to require fat grafting and the techniques for doing so can improve the plastic surgeon's ability to provide optimal aesthetic results following facial skeletal alterations.

▶ This approach demonstrates the powerful results of facial skeletal deficiencies treated with implants and soft tissue deficiencies treated with fat grafts (replace like with like). As the authors point out, facial form ultimately is determined by how the soft tissue envelope drapes over the underlying skeletal foundation. In patients requiring asymmetric or significant skeletal changes, the overlying soft tissue may appear asymmetric, irregular, or hypoplastic. When subtle surface irregularities are visible or palpable, correcting them through fat grafting is a simple, reproducible procedure with permanent results.

K. A. Gutowski, MD

OnabotulinumtoxinA for the Treatment of a "Gummy Smile"

Suber JS, Dinh TP, Prince MD, et al (Univ of South Florida, Tampa, FL)
Aesthet Surg J 34:432-437, 2014

Background.—Excessive gingival display, or a "gummy smile," is defined as 2 mm or more of gingival exposure upon smiling. Such excessive gingival exposure can be aesthetically unappealing to patients. One factor that contributes to a gummy smile is hyperfunctional lip elevator muscles.

Objectives.—The authors evaluate onabotulinumtoxinA as a safe and minimally invasive treatment for a gummy smile.

Methods.—In this prospective study, 14 patients (13 women, 1 man) underwent pretreatment photographs and measurements, followed by bilateral injection of onabotulinumtoxinA into their lip elevator muscles. All patients selected for the study had more than 2 mm of gingival show and were classified as having a "cuspid smile," where action of all elevator muscles raised the upper lip—like a window shade—to expose the upper teeth and gingival scaffold; these patients were thought to have a better chance for a more superior result. Repeat measurements and photographs were collected at 2 weeks and 3 months. Patient-reported outcomes were collected at 2 weeks, and data were compared to determine the correlative relationship.

Results.—An average of 5 units (range, 4-6 U) of onabotulinumtoxinA were injected into 3 sites bilaterally. The average preinjection gingival show over the central incisors and canines were 4.89 mm and 4.25 mm, respectively. Postinjection gingival show decreased to an average of 0.75 mm (85% improvement) and 0.74 mm (83% improvement) over the central incisors and canines, respectively. Average follow-up time was 12.6 days. One patient felt the resulting smile was unattractive and opted not to undergo repeat injections, while all other study participants experienced no negative effects and wished to undergo repeat treatment.

Conclusions.—As treatment for a "gummy smile," onabotulinumtoxinA provides an effective, minimally invasive, and safe therapy. This treatment option can lead to significant improvement in smile aesthetics with high patient satisfaction.

Level of Evidence.—3.

► Gummy smiles have been treated surgically, but a small amount of injectable neuromodulator can have a dramatic result. Dentists and oral surgeons have been using a similar technique for their patients. The critical part is proper injection landmarks and technique to achieve a symmetric smile.

K. A. Gutowski, MD

Aesthetic Applications of Calcium Hydroxylapatite Volumizing Filler: An Evidence-Based Review and Discussion of Current Concepts: (Part 1 of 2)

Emer J, Sundaram H (UCSF Dermatologic Surgery and Laser Ctr, San Francisco, CA; Sundaram Dermatology, Rockville, MD)

J Drugs Dermatol 12:1345-1354, 2013

Background.—Calcium hydroxylapatite filler (CaHA; Radiesse) is a synthetic, non-animal derived product composed of minerals that occur naturally in bone and teeth. Following its development in the US, initial approval by the US FDA for non-aesthetic indications and CE marking in Europe, it was used off FDA-labeling for aesthetic purposes. Its use has grown further since its FDA approval in 2006 for long-lasting correction of moderate to severe wrinkles and folds. It is a popular filler for volume restoration to the face, and also to nonfacial areas such as the dorsum of the hands.

Methods.—The first article of this two-part series provides an evidence-based review of study data pertaining to the mechanism of action and biocompatibility of CaHA filler, and its safety, efficacy and tolerability when used for aesthetic purposes. The review includes data from a number of prospective, controlled comparative studies, from several retrospective studies, and from a meta-analysis of reported complications from alloplastic filler procedures over a 20-year period. The study methodology and number of study subjects are sufficiently robust to provide a high Evidence Level for much of the data.

Results.—CaHA has good safety, efficacy and tolerability profiles that are comparable to those of hyaluronic acid (HA) fillers. It provides an initial, immediate volume replacement for up to 12 months followed by longer term correction due to biostimulation, resulting in collagenesis. Evidence Level II studies show longevity of 30 months or more after nasolabial fold implantation. Other studies demonstrate the appropriateness of CaHA filler for volume restoration to areas including the mid face, lower face and hands. CaHA is classified as an adjustable filler, whereas HA is fully reversible by hyaluronidase digestion. For this reason, and also because of CaHA's high viscosity and elasticity, evidence-based and experiential consensus suggests its avoidance in highly mobile areas (e.g. lips) or in anatomically unforgiving areas (e.g. the periocular region), where there may be increased incidence of nodules.

Conclusion.—CaHA filler is safe, efficacious and well-tolerated when used appropriately. It is increasingly recognized that many patients require pan-facial volume restoration, and that many can benefit from combined treatments. Therefore, CaHA and HA fillers may be considered complementary rather than competitive to each other. The second article of this series offers a discussion of product characteristics, scientific principles and injection techniques to optimize treatment with CaHA filler, including special considerations for avoidance and management of complications.

▶ Most plastic surgeons who use injectable fillers are comfortable with the hyaluronic acids (HAs), Restylane and Juvederm, which are shorter-acting and reversible with hyaluronidase. Calcium Hydroxylapatite (CaHA), Radiesse, is less commonly used, perhaps because of its longer duration of effect, lack of reversibility, and incomplete understanding of its ideal applications among surgeons. Unlike the HA filers, CaHA is a powerful volumizing agent that also stimulates collagen synthesis. Among the current Food and Drug Administration–approved products, it is considered to have the highest G′ (stiffness) making it ideal for lifting tissue, but not for filling in fine lines or augmenting lips. Plastic surgeons interested in expanding their filler product treatment options should review this article.

K. A. Gutowski, MD

Efficacy and Safety of IncobotulinumtoxinA for the Treatment of Platysmal Bands of the Aging Neck: An Open-Label, Prospective Pilot Study

Gubanova EI, Panova OS, Sanchez EA, et al (Vallex M, Clinic of Preventive Medicine, Moscow, Russia; Eclan, Med Ctr of Cosmetological Correction, Moscow, Russia)

J Drugs Dermatol 12:1461-1466, 2013

Introduction.—IncobotulinumtoxinA (Xeomin®/Xeomeen®/Bocouture®/XEOMIN Cosmetic™; botulinum toxin type A, free from complexing proteins [150 kDa], NT 201; Merz Pharmaceuticals GmbH, Frankfurt, Germany) is an effective and well-tolerated treatment for a variety of facial wrinkles.

Objective.—To determine the efficacy and safety of incobotulinumtoxinA for the treatment of platysmal bands.

Methods.—Women, 35–65 years of age, with platysmal bands scoring 2 or 3 on the validated 5-point Merz dynamic platysmal bands scale received a total of 60 U incobotulinumtoxinA divided between four platysmal bands (20 U in both medial bands and 10 U in both lateral bands). Investigator assessments according to the 5-point scale were made at baseline and from standardized clinical photographs taken at follow-up visits 14 ± 2, 56 ± 7 and 84 ± 7 days after treatment. The global aesthetic improvement scale (GAIS) and a novel questionnaire were used to assess subject treatment satisfaction. Adverse events were recorded.

Results.—Twenty-five women (mean age 51.8 years) were included in the study. With a responder defined as a subject with at least a 1-point improvement from baseline on the dynamic platysmal bands scale, the response rate at maximum contraction was 100% at Day 14 as assessed by the investigator. By the same definition, a high response rate (96%) was maintained at maximum contraction at Day 84. Subjects reported that, at Day 84, 86.3% of the maximal effect (defined as the effect on Day 14) persisted. Subject-reported satisfaction was high, as indicated by the self-assessment on the GAIS and results from the subject satisfaction questionnaire. Treatment- related adverse events were mild and reversible.

Conclusion.—IncobotulinumtoxinA is an effective, well-tolerated treatment for platysmal bands, with a high percentage of the treatment effect maintained at 3 months after treatment. Investigator and subject assessments both indicated high levels of treatment satisfaction.

► Although not an FDA-approved indication, botulinum toxins may be used to improve active platysmal bands. Past experience has shown that onabotulinumtoxinA (Botox) may be used for this purpose in 4 to 5 unit injections about 1 to 2 cm apart on each platysmal band. This article reports that incobotulinumtoxinA (Xeomin) may also be used for the same purpose in near the same way with results lasting up to 3 months. Because incobotulinumtoxinA is frequently sold for a lower price than onabotulinumtoxinA, there may be a price advantage to using it if the results are the same as for onabotulinumtoxinA.

K. A. Gutowski, MD

Changing Role of Hyaluronidase in Plastic Surgery

Bailey SH, Fagien S, Rohrich RJ (Univ of Texas Southwestern Med Ctr, Dallas, TX)

Plast Reconstr Surg 133:127e-132e, 2014

Soft-tissue augmentation has become an increasingly popular option for facial rejuvenation. Hyaluronic acid fillers are part of the most rapidly expanding segment of this market, largely because of their safe drug profile and temporary nature. Despite their good safety profile, they can and do have complications ranging from superficial placement, uneven placement, granulomatous reactions, and skin necrosis. This article reviews the on- and off-label uses of hyaluronidase and presents several clinical algorithms detailing the effective and safe use of hyaluronidase to manage complications secondary to hyaluronic acid fillers.

► The use of hyaluronidase to dissolve hyaluronic acid (HA) fillers is currently considered off label by the US Food and Drug Administration, but anyone using HA injectable products should have hyaluronidase available in the event of a complication.

For treatment of excess or misplaced HA product or to eliminate the discoloration associated with superficial product injection (Tyndall effect), hyaluronidase is effective and results are typically seen within a few days. Doses have not been standardized, as the different HA products have variable hyaluronidase degradation. A typical starting amount is 5 to 15 units per site repeated in 1 to 2 weeks if needed. For granulomatous reactions, an intralesional injection of 15 to 75 units of hyaluronidase mixed with 1% lidocaine with epinephrine has been recommended. In rare cases of potential tissue necrosis caused by intra-arterial injection, 30 units or more of hyaluronidase should be injected along the course of the artery (along with use of aspirin, nitropaste, and warm packs).

Animal-derived (Vitrase) and human recombinant (Hylenex) hyaluronidase preparations with the human recombinant form are being recommended because of possibly lower allergic reactions rates.

K. A. Gutowski, MD

Safety and Effectiveness of Large Gel Particle Hyaluronic Acid with Lidocaine for Correction of Midface Volume Loss

Bertucci V, Lin X, Axford-Gatley RA, et al (Univ of Toronto, Ontario, Canada; Division of Valeant Pharmaceuticals, Scottsdale, AZ; Complete Healthcare Communications, Inc, Chadds Ford, PA; et al)

Dermatol Surg 39:1621-1629, 2013

Background.—Midface volume loss and contour deficiency are often treated using soft-tissue fillers capable of elevating and supporting facial features.

Objective.—To evaluate the effectiveness and safety of large gel particle hyaluronic acid with 0.3% lidocaine (LGP-HA-L) for the treatment of midface volume loss or contour deficiency.

Methods and Materials.—This 24-week, open-label study recruited adults aged 18 to 65 with bilateral moderate to substantial midface volume loss or contour deficiency (Medicis Midface Volume Scale (MMVS) score 3–4). The primary effectiveness measure was MMVS response (≥1-grade improvement) 8 weeks after treatment according to evaluators blinded to injection volume.

Results.—All enrolled patients ($n = 40$; 85.0% female; mean ± SD age 53.1 ± 7.0 years) completed the study. Mean ± SD injected volume for both sides of the midface was 5.3 ± 2.5 mL. Week 8 MMVS response rates were 97.5% according to blinded evaluators and treating investigators and 90.0% according to patients; week 24 rates were 90.0%, 92.5%, and 82.5%, respectively. Global Aesthetic Improvement Scale response rates were 95.0% to 100.0% throughout the study. Adverse events were reported in 60.0% of patients and were mild or moderate; all resolved by study end and most within 1 week.

Conclusion.—Midface volume loss or contour deficiency may be safely and effectively corrected using LGP-HA-L.

► The hyaluronic acid gel used in this study was Perlane, which has a high G′ (a measure of the gel's firmness) and also a high G″ (a measure of viscous modulus). Both of these physical characteristics are suited for providing volume and structural support—in this case, to lift the malar region. Proper use of injectable fillers for lifting malar tissue, as opposed to filling in lines and wrinkles, includes selecting a high G′ product (Radiesse would be a nonhyaluronic acid alternative) and correct injection technique. The injection zone in this case was landmarked anatomically as inferior to the maxillary prominence; superior to the plane of nasal alae, including the area from the lateral canthus to the medial canthus; and lateral to the nose. Both subcutaneous and supraperiosteal placement may be used. It is important to remember that undertreatment is likely to result in patient dissatisfaction. The mean initial volume used was nearly 4 mL with a mean touch-up volume of almost 2 mL per patient. Therefore, to achieve a clinically significant improvement, the average patient total injection volume was 5.3 mL +/− 2.5 mL. So although the improvements of malar tissue lifting may be dramatic, the amount of product needed, and therefore cost, needs to be explained to the patient.

K. A. Gutowski, MD

A randomized comparison of the efficacy of low volume deep placement cheek injection *vs.* mid- to deep dermal nasolabial fold injection technique for the correction of nasolabial folds

Goodier M, Elm K, Wallander I, et al (Zel Skin & Laser Specialists, Edina, MN; et al)

J Cosmet Dermatol 13:91-98, 2014

Background.—Hyaluronic acid (HA) fillers are FDA approved for improving the appearance of the nasolabial folds. Previous reports on the use of HA for this treatment have focused on injections directly into the location of the desired correction. To our knowledge, a study has not been done evaluating the efficacy of injecting a low volume of HA into the adjacent area of volume loss to correct both volume loss and adjacent lines.

Objective.—The objective of this study was to compare the effectiveness and safety of three HA injection protocols including deep dermal cheek injection, mid- to deep dermal local nasolabial fold injection, and both injections for the correction of nasolabial folds.

Methods.—This was a split-face, randomized study evaluating the use of three injection techniques – (i) deep bolus injection into the mid- to lateral cheek, (ii) local mid- to deep dermal injection into the nasolabial fold, and (iii) both deep injection into the mid- to lateral cheek and local mid- to deep dermal injection into the nasolabial fold – for the treatment of moderate to severe nasolabial folds. Wrinkle severity and Global Aesthetic Improvement Scales were measured before and 4–6 weeks after treatment as assessed by a blinded investigator.

Results.—Patient and physician observations showed improvement both globally and in wrinkle severity score with each technique used with no statistical difference between techniques. Patients showed a slight preference for injection to both the mid- to lateral cheek and nasolabial fold, which was associated with the greatest amount of filler product administered. No serious adverse events were reported.

Conclusion.—Injection of a dermal filler, at low volumes, into either the nasolabial fold or mid- to lateral cheek results in similar improvement to the correction of the nasolabial folds.

▶ Nasolabial folds due to facial fat migration or soft tissue deflation can be treated by direct soft tissue filler injection into the fold (which may make the area appear too "full") or by restoring volume in the upper lateral cheek, over the malar prominence (which may make the cheeks appear too "puffy"). This study found that both approaches, as well as a combined approach, seem to have similar results. In actual practice, however, it is best to assess each patient's individual facial structure to determine the best injection sites. A patient with adequate malar projection may look unnatural after malar injections to treat the nasolabial fold, whereas a patient with loss of malar prominence would certainly see a better esthetic result from an injection to this area. Likewise, a nasolabial line is better treated with a direct injection. It is also important to explain the findings of the facial assessment and treatment plan to the patient so he or she can appreciate the changes after treatment.

K. A. Gutowski, MD

The Role of Hyaluronidase in the Treatment of Complications From Hyaluronic Acid Dermal Fillers

Cavallini M, Gazzola R, Metalla M, et al (Private Practice, Milano, Italy; Dept at IRCCS Policlinico San Donato, Milano, Italy)
Aesthet Surg J 33:1167-1174, 2013

Hyaluronidases, a family of enzymes that are able to degrade hyaluronic acid (HA), are employed in medicine to increase drug diffusion and reverse the effects of HA filler injections. Hyaluronidases are able to dissolve subcutaneous nodules or to correct excessive quantities of injected filler. Knowledge of the use, methods of application, and adverse effects of hyaluronidases is essential for the aesthetic practitioner. Therefore, we performed an extensive review of the available literature from 1928 to 2011 and compared the different enzymes available, recording each author's indications regarding usage and side effects.

▶ Every practitioner who injects hyaluronic-based fillers should have available, and be familiar with, the use of hyaluronidase. Currently, Hylenex (a human recombinant hyaluronidase), is considered less immunogenic and safer than other preparations. In most cases, low doses are injected (10 to 30 units) into nodules and areas of overtreatment. However, in some cases, repeat injections of up to 600 units total have been reported.

K. A. Gutowski, MD

Five Parameters You Must Understand to Master Control of Your Laser/ Light-Based Devices

Farkas JP, Hoopman JE, Kenkel JM (UT Southwestern Med Ctr, Dallas, TX)
Aesthet Surg J 33:1059-1064, 2013

In this article, the authors review basic fundamental principles of light characteristics and their interaction with the target tissue. It is imperative for the practitioner to understand these concepts to deliver appropriate, efficacious, and safe phototherapeutic treatment for their patients. Once a diagnosis is made and a laser is chosen as a treatment tool, a basic knowledge and understanding of the physics and properties of light/tissue interaction is essential to allow practitioners to provide their patients with optimal results.

▶ A summary of this report will not give the reader the full benefit of actually reading and understanding the concepts described. However, it is worthwhile to at least understand the basics of the 5 parameters discussed.

- The first parameter, wavelength, is determined by the target chromophore (melanin, hemoglobin, oxyhemoglobin, or water). For each wavelength, 2 principles are involved in light-tissue interaction: absorption and scatter. The higher the absorption and the less scatter, the less energy will be required to heat the target to the desired temperature and to achieve the resultant effect. Also, the higher the absorption, the more superficial is the penetration.
- Next, power and spot size are individual parameters that together yield power density, which then determines the amount of energy and heat delivered to the desired target. A change in spot size will also change the depth of penetration, as a smaller spot size will create a more superficial treatment effect. So in general, a decrease in the spot size by half will be needed to deliver double the energy to create an effect at the same treatment depth.
- Pulse width is the energy exposure time of the target tissue and is determined by tissue thermal relaxation time.
- Selective tissue cooling can reduce undesired thermal injury to the epidermis when targeting deeper chromophores (superficial vessels, hair shaft, or dermal water).

For those wishing a better understanding of light-based therapies, this report is required reading.

K. A. Gutowski, MD

Complications in Cosmetic Laser Surgery: A Review of 494 Food and Drug Administration Manufacturer and User Facility Device Experience Reports

Zelickson Z, Schram S, Zelickson B (Univ of Minnesota, Minneapolis; Zel Skin & Laser Specialists, Edina, MN)

Dermatol Surg 40:378-382, 2014

Background.—Complications in cosmetic laser and energy based surgery affect a number of patients every year and may cause scars, burns, blisters, and pigmentation damage.

Objective.—To evaluate documented complications in cosmetic laser- and energy-based surgeries, determine the most common errors, and recommend a simple procedural sequence to reduce patient complications.

Materials and Methods.—U.S. Food and Drug Administration Manufacturer and User Facility Device Experience Adverse Event Reports after cosmetic laser- and energy-based procedures with varied devices were reviewed (N = 494). The laser manufacturer, device used, event type, injury type, cause, operator, and indication for treatment for each case were identified.

Results.—In the 494 cases reviewed between 2006 and 2011, the most common complications were burns, scarring, blistering, pigmentation damage, and infection. The most common cause of these complications was user error by a healthcare provider (30%), followed by laser device malfunction (20%) and patient error (4%). Indications for treatment were unknown for 69% of cases, and 38% of the cases were an unknown cause of complication.

Conclusions.—User error was a major factor in laser surgery complications. To improve safety and reduce errors, we propose the implementation of a procedural sequence for cosmetic laser surgery.

► Not surprisingly, almost one-third of adverse laser and energy device adverse effects were due to user error. Based on this analysis, a safety protocol is recommended staring with a pre-procedure "time out" consisting of verification of patient name, signed consent, treatment site, and device, review of possible contraindications, review of any changes in medications or allergies, confirmation of energy treatment parameters and device settings, environmental check for fire hazards, and use of protective eyewear (when indicated). During the treatment, the medical provider should assess the tissue response after the first pulse and make changes if the response if not appropriate. Pain assessments should be done regularly and treatment stopped if the pain level is too high. Aftercare products and instructions should be confirmed with the patient. It is also wise to make a follow-up phone call the next day to check for any problems.

K. A. Gutowski, MD

Evaluation of microfocused ultrasound with visualization for lifting, tightening, and wrinkle reduction of the décolletage

Fabi SG, Massaki A, Eimpunth S, et al (Goldman Butterwick, Fitzpatrick, Groff, and Fabi, Cosmetic Laser Dermatology, San Diego, CA; Univ of California, San Diego; et al)

J Am Acad Dermatol 69:965-971, 2013

Background.—Laxity and rhytides are manifestations of photodamage on the chest.

Objective.—We sought to evaluate efficacy and safety of microfocused ultrasound with visualization treatment of décolletage laxity and rhytides.

Methods.—In all, 24 subjects with moderate to severe rhytides, as measured by a validated 5-point photonumeric scale (Fabi/Bolton Chest Wrinkle Scale), received microfocused ultrasound with visualization treatment. Efficacy was measured at 90 and 180 days by the Fabi/Bolton Chest Wrinkle Scale, mid-clavicular to nipple distance, masked assessment, Physician and Subject Global Aesthetic Improvement Scales, and patient satisfaction. Adverse events were recorded.

Results.—Rhytides improved over time ($P < .0001$), with 46% and 62% of subjects showing a 1- to 2-point improvement at days 90 and 180, respectively. Mean (SD) mid-clavicular to nipple distance decreased ($P < .0001$), from 20.9 (1.57) cm to 19.8 (1.50) cm and 19.5 (1.59) cm, at days 90 and 180, respectively. At day 90, 100% were improved by Subject Global Aesthetic Improvement Scale score ($P < .0001$) and 96% were improved by Physician Global Aesthetic Improvement Scale score ($P < .0001$), with similar findings at day 180. All subjects were satisfied or very satisfied at day 90, with similar results at day 180. Improvement by masked assessment at day 90 was 71%.

Limitations.—Single-center study, small sample size, and only Fitzpatrick skin types I and II enrolled were limitations.

Conclusion.—There was appreciable efficacy and patient satisfaction after a single microfocused ultrasound with visualization treatment in wrinkle reduction and lifting of the décolletage.

▶ Aging of the upper chest skin, commonly accelerated by sun exposure, is noticed frequently after a patient rejuvenates their facial skin. Unlike the face, aggressive resurfacing is not done in this area, as the skin is thinner, and there are fewer pilosebaceous units for re-epithelialization. Moderate trichloroacetic acid peels, injected poly-L-lactic acid (Sculptra), and fractional lasers have been used to address the aging décolletage. Microfocused ultrasound scan (Ulthera) creates fractional zones of coagulation in the deeper dermis causing collagen tightening and synthesis and is primarily indicated for tightening of neck and facial skin.

It is somewhat hard to interpret the results of this study, as all patients were satisfied with the results, but only 71% of masked evaluators noted improvement. Given that there is no option for rejuvenating the décolletage that delivers consistent results, this device may be offered to patients as long as the limitations are understood.

K. A. Gutowski, MD

Novel Nonablative Radio-Frequency Rejuvenation Device Applied to the Neck and Jowls: Clinical Evaluation and 3-Dimensional Image Analysis

Chipps LK, Bentow J, Prather HB, et al (Moy-Fincher-Chipps Med Group, Beverly Hills, CA; Harbor-UCLA Med Ctr, Torrance, CA; Univ of Pittsburgh, PA)

J Drugs Dermatol 12:1215-1218, 2013

Objective.—To use 3D photography to evaluate the clinical efficacy of a novel radiofrequency delivery device used to improve the appearance of rhytids and laxity of the face and neck.

Study Design.—Forty-nine subjects received a total of two radiofrequency treatments to the face and neck one-month apart. The novel radio-frequency delivery device was used to heat the dermis between 41-43°C for five heat cycles. Primary outcome measures were clinical efficacy quantified by the Global Assessment Improvement Scale (GAIS) and a patient survey that assessed treatment satisfaction.

Results.—Assessments of 3D photographs revealed an overall improvement in 74% of study subjects. 85% of patients noted an overall improvement in the appearance of their skin. 81% of patients rated their post-treatment skin laxity as improved, 85% rated their skin smoothness as improved and 62% rated their skin brightness as improved.

Conclusion.—Subjects in this study demonstrated an overall improvement in face and neck appearance with regard to skin tightening, wrinkles, and skin texture suggested by overall patient satisfaction (85%) and physician-rated GAIS improvement (74%). This study suggests that radiofrequency applied with a continuous thermal treatment device is a safe and efficacious way to improve the overall appearance of aging facial skin.

▶ The jowls and neck laxity are difficult to treat with nonsurgical techniques. Fillers in the prejowl space may camouflage mild jowls, and neuromodulators may soften platysmal bands, but often the underlying skin laxity does not allow for a significant improvement. Pelleve, a nonablative monopolar radiofrequency (RF) device, is one of many RF devices that uses external energy to deliver heat to skin and subcutaneous tissue. This results in collagen molecule tightening and new collagen synthesis with results typically seen in 3 to 6 months. This study showed a modest improvement using standardized 3-dimensional imaging. In clinical use, however, not all patients respond to RF treatment, and expectations must be set regarding the degree of improvement.

K. A. Gutowski, MD

Eyelid

Can topical EMLA cream be used safely in upper blepharoplasty?

Saariniemi KM, Salmi AM, Kuokkanen HO (Vaasa Central Hosp, Finland; Plastic Surgery Clinic KL, Helsinki, Finland; Tampere Univ Hosp, Finland)

Eur J Plast Surg 36:485-488, 2013

Background.—The application of a topical anesthetic eutectic mixture of lidocaine and prilocaine cream (EMLA) has been demonstrated as a simple method to reduce injection pain. However, the use of EMLA near the eye is not recommended in order to avoid accidental corneal irritation or abrasion. We sought to evaluate its effects on immediate and early complications as well as possible adverse reactions in upper blepharoplasty performed under local infiltrative anesthesia.

Methods.—This retrospective case-controlled study consisted of 88 consecutive patients. Fifty-one patients had topical 5 % EMLA administered 15 min before the operation. Thirty-seven patients did not receive topical EMLA and hence comprise the control group. All procedures were performed under local anesthesia by the same surgeon. Possible complications and adverse reactions were recorded at 1 week and 3 months.

Results.—The groups did not differ significantly in respect to the amount of lipectomy performed, postoperative swelling or bruising, wound healing, scar appearance, or corrective procedures. However, surprisingly some more eye irritation, inflammation, or infection was noted in the control group ($p = 0.03$). Overall, a total of eight (9 %) patients had clinically significant bruising, partial wound dehiscence, or conjunctivitis. All resolved with conservative measures.

Conclusions.—The administration of topical EMLA offers a safe and a simple way to complement local infiltrative anesthesia in upper blepharoplasty without increased risk for complications or adverse reactions.

Level of Evidence.—Level III, prognostic/risk study.

▶ According to the authors, the answer is yes, but with some caveats. This is, of course, a nonrandomized study and, as such, is acknowledged by the authors. Furthermore, the authors are very careful with the application of the eutectic mixture of lidocaine and prilocaine (EMLA) cream. EMLA was applied only with patients in the supine position, at least 5 mm from the lash line, and with care taken to avoid its accidental application to the cornea. The cream remained on the eyelid for only 15 minutes. By virtue of the use of EMLA, the authors were able to eliminate the use of sedatives during the course of blepharoplasty and found good results with no long-term complications when compared with the control group. It would be helpful to have this study replicated by others and in a randomized manner.

S. H. Miller, MD

Face, Neck and Brow

Evaluation of Photographic Variables in Patients with Indication for Facial Rejuvenation

Scomação IR, Graf RM, Maluf I Jr, et al (Hospital de Clinicas da, Curitiba, Brazil; Hospital de Clinicas, Curitiba, Brazil; et al)

Aesthetic Plast Surg 37:1114-1119, 2013

Background.—Photography standardization is paramount for appropriate critical analysis of aesthetic surgery outcomes. Therefore, the authors designed a study to evaluate the influence of different variables in photos of patients with indications for undergoing facial rejuvenation.

Methods.—This blinded prospective study was conducted by the Section of Plastic Surgery in the Hospital das Clínicas at the Federal University of Paraná. In the study, 29 patients had their photos taken in two separate settings. Photo 1, termed "preoperative" (Pre), was obtained according to the same pattern for all patients. Photo 2, termed "postoperative" (Post), was acquired on the same day using different variables to manipulate the photo outcome. No surgery was actually performed. Both photos (Pre and Post) were sent to five experienced Brazilian plastic surgeons, who provided a score for photo 2 that varied from −10 to +10 compared with photo 1.

Results.—The photos were examined by 119 plastic surgeons. No significant improvement was observed in most of the groups, except for the group that used a flash for the Post photography ($p = 0.035$). Almost half of the scores (45.37 %) were above zero. The highest score was found to be ten for two photographs of the makeup group. A score of zero was assigned to 54.62 % of the photos, which means no changes occurred between the Pre and Post photos.

Conclusion.—Inadequate photographic technique can change assessments of photos in a meaningful way. All the factors evaluated had a positive impact, but the only statistically significant variable was the use of a flash in the Post group.

Level of Evidence II.—This journal requires that authors assign a level of evidence to each article. For a full description of these Evidence-Based Medicine ratings, please refer to the Table of Contents or the online Instructions to Authors www.springer.com/00266.

▶ Most plastic surgeons can spot false post-treatment improvements in patient images when different photographic techniques are used in the before and after pictures. However, in one of this study's subset of patients, almost half of plastic surgeons judged an improvement in the after pictures when no treatment was done. Proper photographic technique is not only important to assess a surgeon's own results but also for pretreatment planning, especially in facial procedures. Improper lighting and subject distance can make it difficult to make a proper assessment of facial features and landmarks. A review of this article is suggested for those who need to improve their patient imaging.

K. A. Gutowski, MD

Outcomes Assessment of Combination Face Lift and Perioral Phenol–Croton Oil Peel

Ozturk CN, Huettner F, Ożturk C, et al (Cleveland Clinic, OH; Univ of Buffalo, NY)
Plast Reconstr Surg 132:743e-753e, 2013

Background.—Face-lift surgery when combined with perioral phenol–croton oil peel is an underappreciated tool for face rejuvenation. The procedure results in significant central face skin tightening and wrinkle reduction.

Methods.—A retrospective review of 47 consecutive patients who underwent simultaneous face lift and perioral peel was performed. The objective measures used to evaluate the change in appearance of the patients included (1) a validated patient satisfaction questionnaire, (2) an evaluation of apparent age, and (3) an evaluation of perioral wrinkles by independent reviewers using a validated model. The assessment of apparent age was performed as follows: preoperative and postoperative photographs were shown randomly to six reviewers, who were asked to estimate the patient's age. The apparent age was compared with the patient's actual age, and the reduction in apparent age was calculated. Improvement in perioral rhytides was evaluated by using the Glogau classification system (range, 1 to 4).

Results.—Survey results documented overall patient satisfaction, which was rated as 6.5 on a scale of 1 to 7 (with higher scores indicating greater satisfaction). Patients' postoperative apparent age estimate was 8.2 years younger than their real age ($p = 0.0002$). The Glogau classification system score demonstrated a mean reduction of 1.15 (3.3 preoperatively as compared with 2.15 postoperatively, $p < 0.0001$).

Conclusion.—Outcomes measurements, including patient satisfaction, objective evaluation of wrinkle improvement, and significant reduction in apparent age, document the power of this technique.

Clinical Question/Level of Evidence.—Therapeutic, IV.

▶ When considering facial rejuvenation, a facelift alone is often not enough to produce a more youthful appearance. Volume restoration with fat grafting and skin resurfacing can result in a much more dramatic and balanced result when done in combination with a facelift. Improvement in the perioral region is particularly challenging, as it does not respond to facial tissue tightening. For light skinned patients, including a phenol peel is a fast and inexpensive way to improve the outcome without adding additional downtime after the procedure. The authors, however, do not recommend this phenol peel in areas of skin undermining, but alternatives such as trichloracetic acid peel or fractional laser may be used with caution.

K. A. Gutowski, MD

The Lipo-Facelift: Merging the Face-Lift and Liposculpture: Eight Years Experience and a Preliminary Observational Study

Pallua N, Wolter T (Univ Hosp of the RWTH, Aachen, Germany)

Aesthetic Plast Surg 37:1107-1113, 2013

Background.—Since the introduction of the classic submucosal aponeurotic system (SMAS) face-lift, the surgical approach to improve the changes of an aging face has evolved, and significant technical improvements have been made. However, several problems still have not been solved satisfactorily. These problems include facial lipodystrophy and changes in skin and skin texture.

Methods.—The Lipo-Facelift procedure consists of facial liposculpturing performed simultaneously with a biplanar, bivectorial SMAS face-lift procedure. The authors analyzed pre- and postsurgical photographs of 12 patients with a Lipo-Facelift after 3 and 12 months and analyzed their charts for complications. Furthermore, O2C measurement was performed to assess improved microcirculation. The longest follow-up period was 8 years.

Results.—The Lipo-Facelift demonstrated very satisfying results. Initial swelling and bruising were seen as well as two cases of wound-healing disorders, but no surgical intervention or revision was needed. The findings show lasting improvement of skin quality and a youthful appearance.

Conclusion.—The Lipo-Facelift corrects age-related skin and SMAS changes as well as age-related lipodystrophy, improves skin circulation and skin revitalization, and provides a lasting and natural result. The skin quality resulting from simultaneous lipofilling can be explained by improved angiogenesis due to transferred growth factors in the lipoaspirate. Also, differentiation of progenitor cells to fibroblasts and increased production of collagen contribute to firmer skin.

Level of Evidence IV.—This journal requires that authors assign a level of evidence to each article. For a full description of these Evidence-Based Medicine ratings, please refer to the Table of Contents or the online Instructions to Authors www.springer.com/00266.

▶ Restoring facial volume during a facelift procedure is becoming more common. As these authors point out, not just the midface and nasolabial folds can be improved with fat grafts but also the temporal area and the hard-to-treat perioral area and marionette lines. The improvement in facial skin attributed to the fat grafts is consistent with other observations.

K. A. Gutowski, MD

Lift-and-Fill Face Lift: Integrating the Fat Compartments

Rohrich RJ, Ghavami A, Constantine FC, et al (Univ of Texas Southwestern Med Ctr, Dallas; David Geffen School of Medicine at the Univ of California, Los Angeles; Univ of Lyon, France)

Plast Reconstr Surg 133:756e-767e, 2014

Background.—Recent discovery of the numerous fat compartments of the face has improved our ability to more precisely restore facial volume while rejuvenating it through differential superficial musculoaponeurotic system treatment. Incorporation of selective fat compartment volume restoration along with superficial musculoaponeurotic system manipulation allows for improved control in recontouring while addressing one of the key problems in facial aging, namely, volume deflation. This theory was evaluated by assessing the contour changes from simultaneous face "lifting" and "filling" through fat compartment–guided facial fat transfer.

Methods.—A review of 100 face-lift patients was performed. All patients had an individualized component face lift with fat grafting to the nasolabial fold, deep malar, and high/lateral malar fat compartment locations. Photographic analysis using a computer program was conducted on oblique facial views preoperatively and postoperatively, to obtain the most projected malar contour point. Two independent observers visually evaluated the malar prominence and nasolabial fold improvements based on standardized photographs.

Results.—Nasolabial fold improved by at least one grade in 81 percent and by over one grade in 11 percent. Malar prominence average projection increase was 13.47 percent and the average amount of lift was 12.24 percent. The malar prominence score improved by at least one grade in 62 percent of the patients postoperatively, and 9 percent had a greater than one grade improvement. Twenty-eight percent of the patients had a convex malar prominence postoperatively compared with 6 percent preoperatively. Malar prominence improved by at least one grade in 63 percent and by over one grade in 10 percent.

Conclusions.—The lift-and-fill face lift merges two key concepts in facial rejuvenation: (1) effective tissue manipulation by means of lifting and tightening in differential vectors according to original facial asymmetry and shape; and (2) selective fat compartment filling of deep malar and high malar locations and nasolabial fold fat grafting to precisely control facial contouring. This was shown with objective numerical grading and through observer assessment.

Clinical Question/Level of Evidence.—Therapeutic, IV.

► Facial rejuvenation with volume restoration, either using synthetic injectables or autologous fat, is appropriate for a deflated face. In this series, the patients typically had 1 to 3 cc of fat injected into each fat compartment (deep malar, deep medial malar, and high/lateral deep malar fat compartment) and to each nasolabial fold. The standardized before and after images showed improvement in malar shape and projection. This additional step should be considered for most facial rejuvenation procedures where there is an element of volume loss.

K. A. Gutowski, MD

A Novel Approach to Structural Facial Volume Replacement

Sadick NS, Manhas-Bhutani S, Krueger N (Cornell Univ, NY; Sadick Res Group, NY; Univ of Hamburg, Germany)

Aesthetic Plast Surg 37:266-276, 2013

Improved understanding of the anatomy and physiology of the aging face has laid the foundation for adopting an earlier and more comprehensive approach to facial rejuvenation, shifting the focus from individual wrinkle treatment and lift procedures to a holistic paradigm that considers the entire face and its structural framework. This article presents an overview of a comprehensive method to address facial aging. The key components to the reported strategy for improving facial cosmesis include, in addition to augmentation of volume loss, protection with sunscreens and antioxidants; promotion of epidermal cell turnover with techniques such as superficial chemical peels; microlaser peels and microdermabrasion; collagen stimulation and remodeling via light, ultrasound, or radiofrequency (RF)-based methods; and muscle control with botulinum toxin. For the treatment of wrinkles and for the augmentation of pan-facial dermal lipoatrophy, several types of fillers and volumizers including hyaluronic acid (HA), autologous fat, and calcium hydroxylapatite (CaHA) or injectable poly-L-lactic acid (PLLA) are available. A novel bimodal, trivector technique to restore structural facial volume loss that combines supraperiosteal depot injections of volume-depleted fat pads and dermal/subcutaneous injections for panfacial lipoatrophy with PLLA is presented. The combination of treatments with fillers; toxins; light-, sound-, and RF-based technologies; and surgical procedures may help to forestall the facial aging process and provide more natural results than are possible with any of these techniques alone.

Level of Evidence V.—This journal requires that authors assign a level of evidence to each article. For a full description of these Evidence-Based Medicine ratings, please refer to the Table of Contents or the online Instructions to Authors www.springer.com/00266.

▶ For many patients with moderate-to-advanced facial aging, a single treatment modality (neuromodulator, filler, skin care, and resurfacing) is not enough to provide a balanced and natural youthful appearance. The combination of skin protection, muscle control, volume replacement (with multiple products), collagen stimulation, and tissue tightening can offer a blended and dramatic nonsurgical rejuvenation. These concepts are worthwhile to explore for anyone wishing to advance their nonsurgical treatments.

K. A. Gutowski, MD

Three-dimensional soft tissue change after paranasal augmentation with porous polyethylene

Kwon T-G, Kang S-M, Hwang H-D (Kyungpook Natl Univ, Daegu, Republic of Korea)

Int J Oral Maxillofac Surg 43:816-823, 2014

The aim of this study was to investigate the effect of porous polyethylene (PPE) in paranasal augmentation on midfacial soft tissue architecture. This retrospective study recruited patients with midface retrusion and mandibular prognathism. Twenty adult patients who had undergone bilateral PPE augmentation (ready-made type, thickness 4.5 mm, Medpor) to the piriform aperture and simultaneous mandibular setback surgery were included in this study. The soft tissue morphology and thickness of the midface were evaluated using three-dimensional reformatted images from cone beam computed tomography done before and 6 months after surgery. The soft tissue outline of the midface was augmented 1–4 mm. The average increase in soft tissue outline near the peri-alar region was 3.1–3.4 mm, which comprised 68–74% of the PPE thickness ($P < 0.01$). The nasolabial angle and columellar inclination were increased significantly (2.2° and 1.4°, respectively; both $P < 0.05$), whereas the nasal tip angle, nasal tip protrusion, columellar length, and bilateral nostril axis angle did not change. The alar base became wider on average by 2.2 mm ($P < 0.01$). The results showed that paranasal augmentation with PPE significantly increased the overlying soft tissue outline without influencing the nasal projection and could enhance paranasal aesthetics with minimal morbidity.

▶ Midfacial deficiencies due to a concavity around the piriform aperture can cause a "dish-shaped" facial profile, acute nasolabial angle, and a deep groove in the subnasal area. Skeletal procedures (Le Fort I osteotomy, malar osteotomy, or a combination of the 2) can be used to improve severe midface retrusion. For mild or moderate cases, however, augmentation with grafts or implants is possible. This study demonstrated the expected soft tissue projection after implant paranasal augmentation. Although nasal projection may not increase, patients should be informed about the possibility of an increase in the alar base width after surgery.

K. A. Gutowski, MD

Anatomic Evaluation of the Vertical Face-lift in Cadavers

Siwani R, Friedman O (Mayo Clinic, Rochester, MN; Univ of Pennsylvania, Philadelphia)

JAMA Facial Plast Surg 15:422-427, 2013

Importance.—This study investigates how different orientations of tension vectors affect the amount of soft-tissue lift in specific cervicofacial regions.

Objectives.—To compare differences in cosmetic neck and face changes generated by 3 different face-lift techniques, to quantify the amount of lift across different points on the face, and to quantify changes in platysmal dehiscence in each of 3 standard superficial musculoaponeurotic system plication face-lift techniques applied to fresh-frozen cadaver heads.

Design, Setting, and Participants.—Ten cadaver heads in an academic tertiary care center.

Intervention(S).—Three different superficial musculoaponeurotic system plication rhytidectomy procedures were conducted in the following sequence: (1) vertical tension vector plication (vertical lift), (2) superolateral tension vector plication (superolateral lift), and (3) superolateral tension vector plication combined with midline platysmal plication (superolateral lift with platysmal plication).

Main Outcomes and Measures.—After completion of each technique, the amount of lift at 4 standard key points was measured and recorded, and differences in lift at the key points were analyzed.

Results.—Vertical lift was associated with greater total lift than superolateral lift alone or superolateral lift with platysmal plication ($P < .001$ for both). Platysmal dehiscence increased from baseline measurements after superolateral lift and decreased after vertical lift ($P = .002$ for both).

Conclusions and Relevance.—Our findings establish how different orientations of tension vectors applied during face-lift surgery achieve different structural changes to various key points across the face. This study helps the face-lift surgeon and student understand the underlying structural anatomic changes associated with different face-lift techniques, which ultimately result in different cosmetic outcomes.

Level of Evidence.—NA.

▶ Despite the limitations of this cadaver study, the conclusions should be considered when evaluating superficial musculoaponeurotic system (SMAS) elevation vectors. The finding that the lateral tension vector had the best lift suggests that the traditional superior lateral vector may not be ideal, especially when it contributes to platysmal plication dehiscence. In fact, the findings suggest that adding a platysmal plication to an SMAS facelift may need to be reconsidered, as the upward pull on the facial tissue provided by the vertical lift caused apposition of the platysmal edges. The opposing vectors in a superior lateral vector lift combined with a platysmal plication may, in fact, counteract the lifting effects. One unanswered question is the effect of the vector on the nasolabial fold, as this was not measured.

K. A. Gutowski, MD

Measuring Outcomes That Matter to Face-Lift Patients: Development and Validation of FACE-Q Appearance Appraisal Scales and Adverse Effects Checklist for the Lower Face and Neck

Klassen AF, Cano SJ, Scott AM, et al (McMaster Univ, Hamilton, Ontario, Canada; Plymouth Univ Peninsula Schools of Medicine and Dentistry, UK; Memorial Sloan-Kettering Cancer Ctr, NY)

Plast Reconstr Surg 133:21-30, 2014

Background.—The FACE-Q is a new patient-reported outcome instrument to evaluate a range of outcomes for patients undergoing any type of facial cosmetic operation, minimally invasive cosmetic procedure, or facial injectable. This article describes the development and validation of FACE-Q scales relevant to face-lift patients.

Methods.—The FACE-Q was developed by following international guidelines for patient-reported outcome instrument development. For outcomes following a face lift, the authors developed five appearance appraisal scales (i.e., Satisfaction with Cheeks, Satisfaction with Lower Face and Jawline, Appraisal of Nasolabial Folds, Appraisal of Area Under the Chin, and Appraisal of the Neck) and an adverse effects checklist. A field test of these scales was performed in a sample of 225 face-lift patients, and were evaluated using both modern and traditional psychometric methods.

Results.—The five FACE-Q appearance appraisal scales were found to be clinically meaningful, reliable, valid, and responsive to clinical change. These findings were supported by Rasch measurement theory analysis (e.g., overall chi-square values of $p \geq 0.18$; Person Separation Index ≥ 0.88). Responsiveness analyses showed that patient scores for facial appearance improved significantly after treatment ($p < 0.001$); changes in scores were associated with moderate effect sizes (range effect size, 0.40 to 0.79; range standardized response mean, 0.37 to 0.69). Traditional psychometric statistics provided further support (e.g., Cronbach's alpha values $\geq$0.94)

Conclusions.—The FACE-Q appearance appraisal scales are scientifically sound and clinically meaningful and can be used with the adverse effects checklist to measure patient-reported outcomes following a face lift.

▶ The FACE-Q is a validated patient-reported outcomes tool that is similar to the BREAST-Q (a tool used to measure outcomes of breast surgery). For any surgeon considering tracking his or her results (and all should), the FACE-Q should be incorporated into practice to get a better understanding of how patients rate their facelift results.

K. A. Gutowski, MD

The Impact of Endoscopic Brow Lift on Eyebrow Morphology, Aesthetics, and Longevity: Objective and Subjective Measurements over a 5-Year Period

Jones BM, Lo SJ (King Edward VII Hosp, London, UK)

Plast Reconstr Surg 132:226e-238e, 2013

Background.—The longevity of a brow lift, its morphology, and its contribution to overall facial aesthetics have not been addressed in previous studies using both objective measurements and validated subjective aesthetic scoring systems.

Methods.—Thirty-one patients with a 5.4-year follow-up after subperiosteal endoscopic brow lift were assessed by (1) objective measurements using computer software, (2) validated regional aesthetic scoring systems, and (3) global aesthetic scoring systems.

Results.—In part 1, objective measurements confirm a subtle elevation of the brows at less than 5 mm ($p < 0.001$) that persisted at 5.4 years after surgery in all areas except the tail of the eyebrow. In part 2, subjective regional aesthetic scoring indicated that the dimensional change is small but apparent to observers, and is maintained at 5.4 years; that depressor muscle resection with a brow lift provides a statistically significant reduction in glabellar lines, which is maintained at 5.4 years; and that a brow lift provides temporary improvement in forehead lines but that this improvement relapses to baseline at 5.4 years. In part 3, global aesthetic scores suggest that 64 percent patients are still judged as appearing better 5.4 years after a brow lift than before surgery.

Conclusions.—This is the first study to provide evidence from both objective measurements and validated subjective aesthetic scoring systems regarding the morphology, benefits, and longevity of endoscopic brow-lift surgery. This demonstrates that a brow lift produces a subtle elevation, with a natural eyebrow morphology close to the original, and with minimal long-term relapse except at the tail of the eyebrow.

Clinical Question/Level of Evidence.—Therapeutic, IV.

▶ Surgical brow elevation may be less common because of the popularity of neuromodulator injections for brow and forehead aesthetic improvements. Some surgeons find the endoscopic approach less predictable and shorter lasting than an open approach. But even in the endoscopic approach, there is technique variability that may account for suboptimal results. This report suggests that with proper technique, about two-thirds of patients can expect to have results after 5 years that appear better than before surgery, except at the tail of the brow where the results are likely to return to the preoperative position.

K. A. Gutowski, MD

A Failsafe Method to Avoid Injury to the Great Auricular Nerve

Ozturk CN, Ozturk C, Huettner F, et al (Cleveland Clinic, OH; et al)
Aesthet Surg J 34:16-21, 2014

Background.—The great auricular nerve (GAN) is the most commonly injured nerve during facelift surgery. Although rare, injury can result in long-term sequelae.

Objectives.—Previous reports have described the nerve's location at the midbelly of the sternocleidomastoid muscle (SCM) or at its emergence from underneath the SCM. The purpose of our study was to identify the superior course of the great auricular nerve as it applies to facelift.

Methods.—Thirteen fresh cadavers were dissected. A vertical line through the midlobule was drawn perpendicular to the Frankfort's horizontal, acting as a reference to the course of the GAN. Transparent paper overlay tracings were then done to record each nerve's location. The distance from the bony external auditory canal (EAC) to the nerve was measured at the anterior muscle border, at the midbelly of the SCM, and as the nerve emerged from under the SCM. Branching patterns of the nerve and its relation to the external jugular vein were identified.

Results.—In 100% of the dissections, the superior course of the GAN fell within a 30-degree angle constructed using the vertical limb perpendicular to the Frankfurt horizontal and a second limb drawn posteriorly from the midlobule. The distance from the EAC to the nerve was 4.9 ± 1.1 cm at the anterior muscle border, 7.3 ± 1.0 cm at the midbelly of the SCM, and 9.8 ± 1.2 cm at the GAN's emergence from under the SCM. Four types of branching patterns were identified.

Conclusions.—The 30-degree angle described above rapidly and accurately identifies the nerve's location.

▶ This cadaver study adds more information on the location of the great auricular nerve (GAN) and confirms McKinney's original description of the nerve crossing the midbelly of the sternocleidomastoid muscle 7 cm inferior to the external auditory canal. The additional distances should help surgeons be more aware of the GAN location.

K. A. Gutowski, MD

Reducing the Incidence of Hematomas in Cervicofacial Rhytidectomy: New External Quilting Sutures and Other Ancillary Procedures

Neto JC, Rodriguez Fernandez DE, Boles M (Brazilian Society of Plastic Surgery, Vitória, Brazil)
Aesthetic Plast Surg 37:1034-1039, 2013

Background.—Despite the use of many different strategies and techniques and notwithstanding recent advances such as fibrin glue and short scar operations, hematoma remains the most common complication in rhytidectomies.

Methods.—This study analyzed 383 patients who underwent cervicofacial rhytidectomies between September 2006 and March 2012. The patients were distributed into three groups.

Results.—Group 1 comprised patients who had classic face-lifts with epinephrine in the anesthetic solution used to infiltrate the face and neck. The incidence of hematomas in this group was 12 % (24 of 200 patients). Group 2 comprised patients who underwent face-lifts without epinephrine in the solution used to infiltrate the midface and neck. The incidence of hematomas in this group was reduced to 3.6 % (3 of 83 patients). Group 3 comprised the remaining 100 patients, who underwent rhytidectomies with internal and external quilting sutures used in conjunction with other ancillary procedures listed in this report. The incidence of hematomas in this group was reduced to 0 %.

Conclusions.—The most important single procedure that reduced hematoma cases to zero in cervicofacial rhytidectomies was the use of quilting sutures in conjunction with other procedures. Furthermore, the use of these sutures did not cause flap ischemia or necrosis, and there was no adverse impact on the quality of the facial rejuvenation.

▶ The 3 patient groups in this retrospective study were not similar, as the group with the highest hematoma rates also had procedures with more extensive dissections. However, this series may confirm a previous finding that facelift surgery without epinephrine injection may have lower hematoma rates. The main difference was the use of about 20 to 30 external quilting sutures on each cheek and neck to secure the skin flap to the superficial musculoaponeurotic system (SMAS) or platysma. The initial appearance of the face was disturbing because of the multiple suture marks, but it resolved after 2 to 4 weeks when the sutures were removed 2 days after surgery. Unlike internal sutures, which have been used for a similar purpose, the external sutures may cause less temporary skin deformity as they are removed as opposed to allowed to be absorbed over a few weeks.

Other techniques used to reduce hematomas include:

1 Avoiding open communication of the lateral neck with the submental region by using a dilator instead of sharp dissection.
2 Use of a short-scar incision with limited postauricular extension.
3 Limited undermining in the posterior cervical and retroauricular regions.
4 Use of a Minimal access cranial suspension lift instead of SMAS dissection.
5 Perioperative blood pressure monitoring and control.
6 Control of postoperative vomiting and agitation.
7 Mild compressive facial dressings for 3 days.

K. A. Gutowski, MD

Randomized, Controlled, Phase 3 Study to Evaluate the Safety and Efficacy of Fibrin Sealant VH S/D 4 s-apr (Artiss) to Improve Tissue Adherence in Subjects Undergoing Rhytidectomy

Hester TR Jr, Shire JR, Nguyen DB, et al (Private Practice in Atlanta, GA; Private Practice in Chattanooga, TN; Private Practice in Beverly Hills, CA; et al)
Aesthet Surg J 33:487-496, 2013

Background.—Suction drains are commonly placed after rhytidectomy to avoid seroma formation that may result from dead spaces between skin layers. Fibrin sealants promote tissue adherence by crosslinking with extracellular matrix proteins, which may reduce the dead space under skin flaps.

Objectives.—The authors evaluate the safety and efficacy of the fibrin sealant (FS) VH S/D 4 s-apr (Artiss; Baxter Healthcare Corp, Deerfield, Illinois), added to standard-of-care (SoC) treatment, in improving flap adherence and reducing dead space in patients undergoing rhytidectomy.

Methods.—Patients with planned facial rhytidectomy were enrolled in this phase 3, prospective, controlled, randomized, patient-blinded, multicenter trial. They received SoC treatment on 1 side of the face and adjunctive FS VH S/D 4 s-apr on the other.

Results.—Seventy-five patients completed the trial. The mean (SD) drainage volume was 7.7 (7.4) mL from the sides treated with sealant and 20.0 (11.3) mL from the SoC-only sides ($P < .0001$). Rates of hematoma and seroma were similar for the 2 treatments, as were changes in postoperative skin sensitivity. Adverse events generally were mild; 2 serious adverse events were reported (wound abscess, dehydration).

Conclusions.—Adjunct use of FS VH S/D 4 s-apr in rhytidectomy was proven safe in this study. It significantly reduced drainage volumes without increasing the incidence of hematoma or seroma, which suggests that it eliminates dead space through improved flap adherence.

Level of Evidence.—2.

▶ Although a drainage reduction from 20 mL to 7 mL is statistically significant, it is not clinically significant, as there were no statistically significant differences in other measured endpoints, except in postoperative edema, which was more favorable in the Artiss group (but this was assessed by nonblinded investigators). Given these findings, it would be hard to justify the use of Artiss based on this study alone. Perhaps further studies will provide more clinically relevant answers.

K. A. Gutowski, MD

Prevention of Earlobe Deformity in Face-Lifting

Coscia J, Huang A, Stevenson TR (Univ of California Davis Health System, Sacramento)

Ann Plast Surg 70:389-391, 2013

"Pixie-ear" deformity is a postrhytidectomy sequela in which the ear lobe is pulled inferiorly. This deformity may be attributed to excessive skin excision inferior to the earlobe, direct suturing of the facial flap to lobule skin, or excessive scarring. When there is increased tension on the earlobe, the otobasion inferius (cephalic attachment point of lobe) migrates from a posterior cephalic position to an anterior caudal position. The authors present an operative technique to prevent pixie-ear deformity and optimize earlobe position in face-lifting.

▶ Preventing earlobe deformity needs to be considered, especially when dealing with an attached earlobe during a facelift. Using this technique, the facelift incision is brought up on the inferior portion of the ear lobe to allow for a wedge defect to be created. Closing this defect then rounds out the earlobe before it is inset.

K. A. Gutowski, MD

The Endonasal Lip Lift: Personal Technique

Raphael P, Harris R, Harris SW (Plastic Surgeons in Private Practice in Plano, TX; Med student at Univ of Texas—Southwestern, Dallas, TX)

Aesthet Surg J 34:457-468, 2014

Given the shortcomings of current methods to shorten the cutaneous upper lip, the senior authors modified the traditional subnasal lip lift with endonasal flaps, performing 311 such lifts over a 15-year period. Ideal surgical candidates are adults with tall philtra, negligible dental show, and no maxillary abnormalities. Benefits of the procedure include improved scar appearance and pout, absence of tension in visible areas, increased dental and vermilion display, and minimal scar migration (ie, loss of lift). Moreover, caudal rhinoplasty procedures are facilitated via the same incision sites. Undercorrection, sill widening, and alar distortion are mostly avoidable (or at least corrigible) complications. Nasal sill disruption, however, remains an inevitable drawback that may be minimized through meticulous technique

▶ The endonasal lip lift was described many years ago and in selected patients can shorten a long upper lip with very minimal scaring. It is not an alternative to lip augmentation (with filler), as the lift everts the labia but does not add volume. The combination of lip lift and lip augmentation is appropriate with a long upper lip and short labial height. A corner lip lift can be considered at the same time to improve a downward slanting commissure. A small dose of neuromodulator can soften the active perioral lines for a more powerful result.

K. A. Gutowski, MD

Surgical Decompression of the Great Auricular Nerve: A Therapeutic Option for Neurapraxia following Rhytidectomy

Barbour JR, Iorio ML, Halpern DE (Georgetown Univ Hosp, Washington, DC; Univ of South Florida, Tampa, FL)

Plast Reconstr Surg 133:255-260, 2014

Background.—Great auricular nerve injuries are the most frequent nerve injuries following rhytidectomy, occurring at a rate of 6 percent. Short-scar techniques may decrease visualization and increase the risk of injury/compression of the great auricular nerve. Recent reviews have identified that great auricular nerve injury can contribute to long-term paresthesias and allodynia in a majority of patients. Identification of this injury, with subsequent exploration, wide release, and decompression, should be performed.

Methods.—Four patients with injury of the great auricular nerve were referred for persistent allodynia as a complication of short-scar rhytidectomy. Following confirmation of a Tinel sign over the great auricular nerve, each patient underwent subsequent exploration and neurolysis.

Results.—Diagnosis of compression and suture impingement was confirmed at exploration, and extensive decompression was performed with care taken to protect the nerve from postoperative scar formation. All patients noted postoperative improvement in symptoms, with nearly complete resolution at 6 months.

Conclusions.—Minimally invasive techniques may impart increased risk of nerve injury in exchange for reduced scar length. In instances of great auricular nerve injury, progressive metabolic changes and increased vascular permeability allow for inflammatory cellular influx and fibrin deposition, compounding nerve dysfunction and symptomatic complaints. Noninvasive modalities may not alleviate complaints of pain and hyperesthesia, particularly in the event of suture compression. Persistent injuries can affect quality of life, with intrusive thoughts about symptoms, or an inability to perform grooming activities. Exploration and decompression of the great auricular nerve may offer a long-term solution for the patient with postrhytidectomy allodynia.

Clinical Question/Level of Evidence.—Therapeutic, V.

▶ Great auricular nerve (GAN) injury is reported in up to 6% of facelifts. In most cases, conservative measures and time will lead to resolution. However, in significant nerve injury, suture compression, or complete transection, a painful neuroma may result. A positive Tinel's sign suggests operative GAN exploration.

If a Tinel's sign is not present, exploration may be warranted if symptoms are not improving after 6 months.

K. A. Gutowski, MD

Nose

Effect of Pregabalin and Dexamethasone Addition to Multimodal Analgesia on Postoperative Analgesia Following Rhinoplasty Surgery

Demirhan A, Tekelioglu UY, Akkaya A, et al (Abant Izzet Baysal Univ Med School, Bolu, Turkey)

Aesthetic Plast Surg 37:1100-1106, 2013

Background.—We investigated the effect of a combination of pregabalin and dexamethasone, when used as part of a multimodal analgesic regimen, on pain control after rhinoplasty operations.

Methods.—Sixty patients were enrolled in this study. They were randomly assigned into three groups: Group C (placebo + placebo), Group P (pregabalin + placebo), and Group PD (pregabalin + dexamethasone). Patients received either pregabalin 300 mg orally 1 h before surgery, dexamethasone 8 mg intravenously during induction, or placebo according to their allocation. Postoperative pain was treated with intravenous patient-controlled analgesia (tramadol, 20-mg bolus dose, 45-min lockout time). The numeric rating scale (NRS), side effects, and consumption of tramadol, pethidine, and ondansetron were assessed.

Results.—The median NRS scores at 0, 1, and 6 h after surgery were significantly higher in Group C than in Group PD ($p < 0.001$ for all). The 24-h consumption of tramadol and pethidine was significantly reduced in Groups P and PD compared to Group C ($p < 0.01$ and $p < 0.01$). The total tramadol consumption was decreased by 54.5% in Group P and 81.9% in Group PD compared to Group C ($p < 0.001$ for both). The incidence of nausea was higher in Group C than in Groups P and PD between the postoperative 0–2 and 0–24-h periods ($p < 0.05$ for both). The frequency of blurred vision was significantly higher in Groups P and PD than in Group C within the 0–24-h period ($p < 0.05$ for both).

Conclusion.—We found that the addition of a single dose of pregabalin and dexamethasone to multimodal analgesia in rhinoplasty surgeries provided efficient analgesia and thus decreased opioid consumption.

Level of Evidence I.—This journal requires that authors assign a level of evidence to each article. For a full description of these Evidence-Based Medicine ratings, please refer to the Table of Contents or the online Instructions to Authors www.springer.com/00266.

▶ Pregabalin, an agent originally developed to treat neuropathic pain, has been recommended as having beneficial effects on perioperative pain. In this nice prospective, double-blinded study, the authors show its effectiveness, alone and when combined with dexamethasone, in ameliorating pain during the first postoperative day after rhinoplasty. The combination of Pregabalin and dexamethasone was more efficacious than Pregabalin alone. It is curious that the authors did not choose to add a fourth study group (placebo + dexamethasone) to the other 3 (placebo + placebo, Pregabalin + placebo, and Pregabalin + dexamethasone). The groups were small, 20 patents in each, and there appeared to be some differences in the male and female participants in each group and differences in the duration of surgery and anesthesia, but these differences did not reach statistical significance. Obviously, further study needs to be done to confirm these findings and to rule out other confounding variables.

S. H. Miller, MD

Inferior turbinate hypertrophy: Review and graduated approach to surgical management

Brunworth J, Holmes J, Sindwani R (Univ of California–Irvine; Cleveland Clinic Foundation, OH)

Am J Rhinol Allergy 27:411-415, 2013

Background.—Surgical techniques for managing inferior turbinate hypertrophy (ITH) vary widely and have evolved substantially in the past four decades as new technologies have emerged.

Methods.—Literature review.

Results.—Inferior turbinate (IT) procedures can be categorized as: simple turbinate outfracture; turbinoplasty techniques such as extramucosal destruction, and submucosal tissue removal; and extramural turbinate resection (partial or complete). Each of these approaches has advantages and drawbacks. Considerations for technique selection include clinical setting (in-office versus operating room), cost of the devices used, efficacy of the procedure to relieve nasal obstruction, and minimizing postoperative complications such as nuisance bleeding, adhesion formation, and crusting.

Conclusion.—There are a variety of contemporary surgical techniques used for IT reduction. This article highlights the available literature and gaps in current knowledge. A graduated approach to the management of ITH will be presented.

▶ Inferior turbinate hypertrophy is common during functional rhinoplasty and is occasionally encountered in aesthetic rhinoplasty. A rational treatment algorithm is important so as not to overtreat the problem and potentially cause complications or other airway compromise. This report is recommended for plastic surgeons who need a concise review of the pros and cons of the available options. The authors suggest that the technique selected should be individualized to the specific clinical situation. Guiding principles based on evidence and trends in the literature suggest:

- All techniques have been shown to offer benefit and improve nasal obstruction
- Surface-sparing techniques appear to have advantages of less crusting, fewer adhesions, and possibly less pain

- Actually removing turbinate tissue submucosally appears to have lasting advantages over less-aggressive techniques
- Extramural turbinate resection removes the maximal amount of tissue but is also associated with the highest morbidity of all techniques
- Multiple techniques (especially outfracture) may be combined to maximize effectiveness

K. A. Gutowski, MD

Inferior Turbinoplasty During Cosmetic Rhinoplasty: Techniques and Trends

Tanna N, Im DD, Azhar H, et al (New York Univ; Univ of California, Los Angeles; Univ of Michigan, Ann Arbor)

Ann Plast Surg 72:5-8, 2014

Background.—The sheer number of accepted inferior turbinoplasty techniques emphasizes the fact that there is no general agreement on which approach yields optimal results, nor are there data available that describes prevalent techniques in turbinate surgery among plastic surgeons.

Objective.—The aim of this study was to identify practice patterns among plastic surgeons who perform inferior turbinoplasty during rhinoplasty.

Methods.—Members of the American Society of Plastic Surgeons were invited to participate in an anonymous, Internet-based survey containing questions related to personal preferences and outcomes in inferior turbinate surgery.

Results.—A total of 534 members of the American Society of Plastic Surgeons participated in the survey. Most (71.7%) trained in an independent plastic surgery program with prerequisite training in general surgery. More than half (50.6%) had more than 20 years of operative experience; only 15.2% reported performing greater than 40 rhinoplasties per year. The 5 most preferred inferior turbinate reduction techniques were outfracture of the turbinates (49.1%), partial turbinectomy (33.3%), submucous reduction via electrocautery (25.3%), submucous resection (23.6%), and electrocautery (22.5%). Fewer than 10% of the respondents reported the use of newer techniques such as radiofrequency thermal ablation (5.6%), use of the microdebrider (2.2%), laser cautery (1.1%), or cryosurgery (0.6%). Mucosal crusting and desiccation were the most frequently reported complications.

Conclusions.—The results of this survey provide insights into the current preferences in inferior turbinate reduction surgery. Plastic surgeons are performing more conventional methods of turbinate reduction rather than taking advantage of the many of the more novel technology-driven methods.

▶ It seems intuitive to most surgeons evaluating a patient for nasal surgery/cosmetic rhinoplasty that evaluation of not only the appearance of the nose but also its function is desirable and mandatory. As such, nasal obstruction, whether caused by septal obstruction, inferior turbinate hypertrophy, or collapse of the nasal vault, all must be evaluated and appropriately diagnosed before undertaking cosmetic rhinoplasty and informing the patient of any premorbid condition that might affect the function of his or her nose after cosmetic rhinoplasty. This study addresses an important subject but adds little in the way of knowledge about the subject. First, the response rate to the survey was very small (10%); most of the respondents (51%) had been in practice less than 5 years, and most did less than 25 rhinoplasties in a year. The authors state that few plastic surgeons utilize the more recent technologic developments for the treatment of inferior turbinate hypertrophy, but it is unclear as to which provide the best outcomes. In light of the small number of plastic surgeons responding to the survey having had exposure to otolaryngology during their training and the fact that most of these newer techniques have been described in the otolaryngology literature, the authors need to explore methods to bring these newer techniques to those plastic surgeons performing significant numbers of cosmetic rhinoplasty. Moreover, multicenter studies need to be conducted to evaluate the techniques, complications, and outcomes of surgery performed for inferior turbinate hypertrophy.

S. H. Miller, MD

The Potential Effects of Rhinoplasty on Voice

Foroughian M, Khazaeni K, Haghi MR, et al (Mashhad Univ of Med Sciences, Iran; Ferdowsi Univ of Mashhad, Iran)

Plast Reconstr Surg 133:109e-113e, 2014

Background.—Rhinoplasty is one of the most popular cosmetic surgical procedures in Iran. Surgery on the vocal tract can potentially change the voice characteristics. To the best of the authors' knowledge, no study has described voice changes after rhinoplasty, and the results of this study may help physicians to be aware of potential voice alterations following rhinoplasty.

Methods.—The authors selected 27 patients for this study. Patients completed Voice Handicap Index questionnaires, and the authors performed perceptual and acoustic analyses before and 5 months after rhinoplasty.

Results.—The Voice Handicap Index score and its physical and emotional subscales showed a statistically significant increase after rhinoplasty, indicating a worsening of voice quality after rhinoplasty. Blind perceptual analysis by six trained listeners revealed a statistically significant increase in hyponasality after rhinoplasty. Acoustic analysis showed that the frequency of the first and second nasal murmurs increased for the phonemes "m" and "n," while the amplitude of these murmurs decreased significantly after surgery. The same pattern was seen for the phoneme "a" when it was produced between two nasal consonants, as in the word "man."

Conclusions.—Rhinoplasty can change vocal characteristics by narrowing the nasal cavity. Rhinoplasty has some effects on the voice, but these changes are problematic in general for most patients. However, for individuals who rely on their voice for professional reasons, the surgeon should preoperatively discuss these changes with the patient and consider more conservative types of surgery.

Clinical Question/Level of Evidence.—Therapeutic, IV.

▶ "Does the voice change after nasal surgery?" is a frequently asked question, and responses are quite varied but rarely based on any evidence whatsoever. Little in the way of objective study and evaluation has been performed before that presented by these authors. Their study seems to show quite clearly that rhinoplasty does result in hyponasality (judged by the patients and blind analysis performed by 6 trained listeners) at least 5 months after the procedure has been performed. Whether these effects will ameliorate, worsen, or stabilize if evaluated during a longer-term follow-up is unknown. Other authors, studying the effects of septoplasty, found no change in voice quality after septoplasty alone.[1] One of the issues that is unclear in my mind is the generalizability of the data as they might relate to the voice quality of individuals singing in languages other than Farsi.

S. H. Miller, MD

Reference

1. Koc E, Koc B, Ercan I, Tadihan E, Turgut S. Effects of septoplasty on speech and voice. *J Voice*. 2013;13:193-198.

Rhinoplasty: Congenital Deficiencies of the Alar Cartilage

Kosins AM, Daniel RK, Sajjadian A, et al (Univ of California, Irvine; Plastic Surgeon in Private Practice in Newport Beach, CA)

Aesthet Surg J 33:799-808, 2013

Background.—Congenital deficiencies of the alar cartilages are rare and often visible at birth but can occasionally present later.

Objectives.—The authors review the anatomical development and discuss the incidence and treatment of congenital defects within the alar cartilages seen in rhinoplasty cases.

Methods.—The charts of 869 consecutive patients who underwent open rhinoplasty were retrospectively reviewed, and 8 cases of congenital defects of the alar cartilage within the middle crura were identified. Intraoperative photographs were taken of the alar deformities, and each patient underwent surgical correction. To simplify analysis, a classification of the defects was developed. A division was a cleft in the continuity of the alar cartilage with the 2 ends separate. A gap was a true absence of cartilage ranging from 1 to 4 mm, which can be accurately assessed in unilateral cases. A segmental loss was a defect greater than 4 mm.

Results.—The 8 cases of deformity could be classified as 4 divisions, 3 gaps, and 1 segmental loss. None of the patients had a history of prior nasal trauma or nasal surgery. Six patients were women and 2 patients were men. In all cases, adequate projection and stability were achieved with a columellar strut. Asymmetry was minimized through concealer or tip grafts. There were no complications.

Conclusions.—Surgeons performing rhinoplasty surgery will encounter and should be prepared to deal with unexpected congenital defects of the alar cartilage. These defects within the middle crura will require stabilization with a columellar strut and, often, coverage with a concealer tip graft. We speculate that the cause of these defects is a disruption of the hedgehog signals that may arrest the condensation or block the differentiation of the underlying neural crest cells.

▶ Congenital alar cartilage deficiencies are rare (1% in this series) and are seldom diagnosed before surgery. Although tip or nostril asymmetry may suggest a congenital deficiency, intraoperative assessment is required. For a simple cartilage division without a gap, the ends of the cartilage are repaired, and a columellar strut is placed. A "concealer graft" of alar cartilage may be used to cover any irregularities or asymmetries. For gaps of 1 to 4 mm, treatment depends on the extent of tip deformity and loss of projection and definition. A major septocolumellar strut may be needed to provide maximum tip support to the tip, and a rigid tip graft can be placed for definition. For a segmental loss of more than 4 mm, the domal junction and columellar breakpoint should be aligned on the 2 sides and an interposition graft of excised alar cartilage be placed to bridge the defect. As in simple division defects, a "concealer graft" can be used to smooth the area. In unilateral cases, the defect side should match the normal side.

K. A. Gutowski, MD

The Sandwiched Lateral Crural Reinforcement Graft: A Novel Technique for Lateral Crus Reinforcement in Rhinoplasty

Kuran İ, Öreroğlu AR (Plastic Surgeon in Private Practice in Istanbul, Turkey; Dr. A. Ilhan Ozdemir State Hosp, Giresun, Turkey)

Aesthet Surg J 34:383-393, 2014

Background.—Misshapen or weak lateral crura can cause an inward collapse of the lateral crus observed on deep inspiration. The lateral crural strut graft is a popular technique for reinforcing lateral crura. Failure to stabilize the graft properly can, however, result in graft displacement postoperatively and an accompanying aesthetic deformity.

Objectives.—The authors discuss lateral crus reinforcement with the sandwiched lateral crural reinforcement (SLCR) graft.

Methods.—An SLCR graft was placed in 30 nonconsecutive primary open-approach rhinoplasty procedures by the senior author (İ.K.) between February 2010 and May 2012. Cephalic excess of the lateral crura was incised and placed under the lateral crura; the lateral crural strut grafts were placed between the 2 cartilages, and the cephalic edges of both the superior and inferior lateral crura segments were sutured together.

Results.—Of the 30 patients, there were 5 men and 25 women ranging in age from 22 to 45 years (median, 35 years). Half (50%) of the patients received the SLCR graft for external valve collapse; in 30% of the patients, it was placed to support the lateral crura after correcting cephalic malpositioning; and 20% had an SLCR graft placed for lateral crural reinforcement after deformity secondary to dome-shaping sutures. No graft displacement or tip disfigurement was observed in the follow-up period (mean, 24 months).

Conclusions.—The SLCR graft technique represents a powerful tool for reinforcing lateral crura without discarding the cephalic portion of the cartilage, thus securing a stable graft pocket while minimizing any postoperative structural dislocation.

Level of Evidence.—4.

▶ Reusing the excised portion of the cephalic lower lateral cartilage has been described; it can be useful to reinforce the remaining cartilage strip and prevent future collapse or deformity. This technique demonstrates the principle and shows how it can be combined with a lateral crus reinforcement graft. A video of this technique may be viewed at http://www.youtube.com/watch?v=kAk8drJJbDM.

K. A. Gutowski, MD

The Deviated Nose and Asymmetric Eyebrows: An Important Trap to Avoid

Katira K, Guyuron B (Univ Hosps Case Med Ctr, Cleveland, OH)

Plast Reconstr Surg 133:519-523, 2014

Background.—Failure to recognize asymmetrically positioned eyebrows, often altered by the patient to camouflage nasal asymmetry, can lead the surgeon to design the rhinoplasty using a faulty midline landmark. The purpose of this study was to investigate the frequency of eyebrow asymmetry and to test whether there is an association between eyebrow position and the direction of nasal deviation.

Methods.—Life-size photographs of 100 rhinoplasty patients were selected randomly from the senior author's (B.G.) practice. Nasal deviation from the midpoint of the intercanthal distance was measured at standardized levels on anteroposterior views corresponding to the nasal bones, upper lateral cartilages, and nasal tip. The maximally deviated parameter was noted.

Results.—Of the 27 men and 73 women studied, 96 patients had measurable eyebrow asymmetry, including 96 percent of men and 96 percent of women. All 100 patients had at least one level of nasal deviation. The direction of eyebrow shift correlated significantly with the direction of nasal deviation for nasal bones ($p = 0.0018$), nasal tip ($p = 0.0032$), and maximally deviated parameter ($p = 0.039$), but not for upper lateral cartilages ($p = 0.54$). Mean eyebrow shift distance for male patients (1.8 mm) and female patients (1.3 mm) was not significantly different ($p = 0.056$).

Conclusions.—The frequency of eyebrow asymmetry and the significant correlation between eyebrow position and nasal deviation direction suggest that eyebrows can camouflage nasal deformities. Furthermore, the alarmingly high incidence of nasal deviation in rhinoplasty candidates emphasizes the value of a circumspect preoperative nasal analysis in reducing the incidence of residual postoperative nose deviation.

Clinical Question/Level of Evidence.—Risk, IV.

▶ Achieving optimal rhinoplasty results requires proper preoperative analysis and avoiding anatomic traps that can cause a misleading analysis. The authors describe a new way in which brow position, when used as a midline reference point, can influence the assessment of a deviated nose.

The eyebrow position may be altered by a patient plucking their brow in an effort to achieve a more symmetric appearance. If this is unrecognized by the surgeon, the preoperative planning may underappreciate the degree of nasal deviation and the rhinoplasty design may be based on an incorrect midline landmark. Alternatively, if the patient is not aware of the eyebrow asymmetry before surgery, they may see a perceived nasal deviation after surgery.

Therefore, the proper facial midline should be used (the vertical line bisecting the intercanthal distance), as it is a reference for facial symmetry in all 3 facial zones (passing through the forehead, upper lip, and chin), and it cannot be manipulated by patients.

K. A. Gutowski, MD

Corrective Nasal Surgery in the Younger Patient

Adil E, Goyal N, Fedok FG (Penn State Milton S. Hershey Med Ctr, PA)

JAMA Facial Plast Surg 16:176-182, 2014

Importance.—To describe clinical parameters for the management of the pediatric patient with nasal anatomical deformity or functional impairment.

Objectives.—To review the authors' experience with corrective nasal surgery in pediatric patients and make recommendations regarding indications for surgery and surgical techniques.

Design, Setting, and Participants.—A retrospective medical chart review was performed for all male patients younger than 16 years and female patients younger than 14 years seen by the senior author (F.G.F.) at a tertiary referral center between August 1996 and August 2012. The database was searched for patients who underwent septoplasty or corrective nasal surgery by the senior author.

Exposures.—Patients included in the study underwent either septoplasty or corrective nasal surgery by the senior author.

Main Outcomes and Measures.—Age, indication for surgery, surgery performed, and last follow-up appointment was recorded for each patient. In addition, any complications or need for revision surgical or adjunct procedures were noted.

Results.—Demographics and outcomes for 54 pediatric patients were included in the study. The most common indications for surgery were post-traumatic deformities (n = 36) and severe airway obstruction (n = 48). Fifteen patients with severe nasal airway obstruction did not have a documented history of trauma. The mean follow-up period was 646 days (approximately 21 months), with a range of 8 to 4062 days. Five patients underwent a staged procedure, and no patients underwent a revision procedure for unsatisfactory results.

Conclusions and Relevance.—Children with nasal obstruction and deformity can safely undergo nasal corrective surgery prior to adolescence. Special considerations include preserving normal structures and the judicious use of grafts. The recommended approaches to managing the pediatric septoplasty and nasal surgery patient are described herein through a series of representative cases.

▶ Functional nasal surgery in preadolescent patients has potential concerns of damage to nasal growth centers with a resulting decrease in nasal ventral and caudal projection. However, in cases of significant deformity or functional issues such as airway obstruction, surgical intervention may be appropriate. Although continued growth and aging may show new deformities, this study suggests that younger patients may benefit from earlier nasal surgery, including the use of cartilage grafts, without subsequent facial growth problems. The main limitation of this series is the short follow-up period of 21 months.

K. A. Gutowski, MD

Septoturbinotomy

Tanna N, Lesavoy MA, Abou-Sayed HA, et al (North Shore-LIJ Health System, Manhasset, NY; Univ of California, Los Angeles; Univ of Miami Miller School of Medicine, FL; et al)

Aesthet Surg J 33:1199-1205, 2013

The inferior turbinates are a principal cause of nasal airway obstruction. To some extent, the bony septum (the perpendicular plate of the ethmoid) also, on occasion, contributes to that airflow obstruction. There are many excellent methods to resect or ablate the turbinates, including submucous resection and cauterization. However, some have been associated with bleeding, crusting, and the development of synechiae. In this Featured Operative Technique article, we propose 2 mechanical means to expand the nasal vault: (1) the insertion of a large and long speculum that outfractures the turbinates and also centralizes the bony septum when the handles are compressed and (2) the insertion of a large clamp, which is expanded (in reverse "nutcracker" fashion) to achieve a similar result. Mechanical dilation (expansion) of the nasal vault with the speculum or large clamp substantially improves vault diameter such that further work on the turbinates in the form of turbinectomy is seldom necessary. The nasal vault is not necessarily expanded to the maximal diameter that could be achieved with resection procedures but need not be to achieve satisfactory air flow. Septoturbinotomy is a quick and simple way to deal with inferior turbinate hypertrophy. It is a minimally invasive procedure that improves the airway in virtually all cases, such that turbinectomy is seldom employed. It can be used prophylactically on all rhinoplasty cases requiring lateral osteotomy, which potentially shrinks the nasal vault slightly.

▶ Instead of turbinate resections, less destructive techniques may be considered to treat inferior turbinate hypertrophy. Turbinate outfracture is a fast and easy maneuver that can be done with a 3-inch nasal speculum. If done properly, it can also improve deflections of the bony septum at the same time. Using cadavers, the authors showed increases in nasal vault diameter of 64%, which results in a theoretical 7-fold increase in airflow.

Refer to the previous article, Inferior Turbinate Hypertrophy: Review and Graduated Approach to Surgical Management, for more on treatment of turbinate hypertrophy.

K. A. Gutowski, MD

Comparison of nasal packs with transseptal suturing after nasal septal surgery

Özkırıs M, Kapusuz Z, Saydam L (Bozok Univ Med Faculty, Yozgat/Turkey)
Am J Otolaryngol 34:308-311, 2013

Objectives.—To investigate the effects of transseptal suturing against two different types of nasal packs with respect to pain, operative time and postoperative complications following nasal septal surgery.

Patients and Methods.—One hundred and fifty patients (aged 18–61 years) scheduled for nasal septal surgery were included. Following surgery, three types of nasal packing systems were utilized: (1) transseptal suturing (Group A: 50 patients); (2) internal nasal splint (Group B: 50 patients); (3) a Merocel standard 8-cm nasal dressing without airway

(Group C: 50 patients) to the patients. Postoperative pain, operation time, septal perforation and synechiae formation were evaluated.

Results.—The difference between mean operative time of groups B and C was not statistically significant ($p > 0.05$). The difference between operative time of the two groups against group A was statistically significant ($p < 0.05$). The mean postoperative pain scores were 2.8 ± 1.2 (median 2) in group A, 6.1 ± 1.3 (median 6) in group B, and 7.3 ± 1.2 (median 7) in group C 1 h to 48 h post-surgery. Merocel and internal nasal splint tampons were found to be significantly more painful than transseptal suturing during 48 h ($p < 0.05$). There was no statistically significant difference in terms of infection, hematoma, synechiae formation or perforation between the groups ($p > 0.05$).

Conclusion.—The use of transseptal suturing technique is a useful alternative to packing, with only minor increase in operating time.

► The authors nicely demonstrate less patient discomfort after using 4 separate 4-0 Vicryl transseptal sutures compared with internal nasal splints or pads, without an increase in complications. Although it adds about 5 minutes to place the sutures, the improvement in patient comfort may be worth the time spent.

K. A. Gutowski, MD

From the Operating Room to the Courtroom: A Comprehensive Characterization of Litigation Related to Facial Plastic Surgery Procedures

Svider PF, Keeley BR, Zumba O, et al (Univ of Medicine and Dentistry of New Jersey; Mount Sinai School of Medicine, NY; et al)

Laryngoscope 123:1849-1853, 2013

Objectives/Hypothesis.—Malpractice litigation has increased in recent decades, contributing to higher health-care costs. Characterization of complications leading to litigation is of special interest to practitioners of facial plastic surgery procedures because of the higher proportion of elective cases relative to other subspecialties. In this analysis, we comprehensively examine malpractice litigation in facial plastic surgery procedures and characterize factors important in determining legal responsibility, as this information may be of great interest and use to practitioners in several specialties.

Study Design.—Retrospective analysis.

Methods.—The Westlaw legal database was examined for court records pertaining to facial plastic surgery procedures. The term "medical malpractice" was searched in combination with numerous procedures obtained from the American Academy of Facial Plastic and Reconstructive Surgery website.

Results.—Of the 88 cases included, 62.5% were decided in the physician's favor, 9.1% were resolved with an out-of-court settlement, and 28.4% ended in a jury awarding damages for malpractice. The mean settlement was $577,437 and mean jury award was $352,341. The most litigated procedures were blepharoplasties and rhinoplasties. Alleged lack of informed consent was noted in 38.6% of cases; other common complaints were excessive scarring/disfigurement, functional considerations, and postoperative pain.

Conclusions.—This analysis characterized factors in determining legal responsibility in facial plastic surgery cases. Several factors were identified as potential targets for minimizing liability. Informed consent was the most reported entity in these malpractice suits. This finding emphasizes the importance of open communication between physicians and their patients regarding expectations as well as documentation of specific risks, benefits, and alternatives.

▶ Communication issues are at the core of most patient safety process breakdowns, are associated with many medical complications, and, as we see in this report, contribute to medicolegal actions. In these cases, more than one-third of legal actions revolved around an alleged lack of informed consent. Common complaints were associated with scaring and disfigurement. The authors appropriately stress the importance of explicitly covering and documenting potential complications in a discussion of risks, benefits, and alternatives with patients, with specific focus on scaring, pain, and potential functional problems after surgery.

K. A. Gutowski, MD

Trunk, Genitalia and Extremities

Outpatient Lipoabdominoplasty: Review of the Literature and Practical Considerations for Safe Practice

Levesque AY, Daniels MA, Polynice A (Albany Med Ctr, NY)
Aesthet Surg J 33:1021-1029, 2013

Background.—Lipoabdominoplasty, popularized by Saldanha et al in 2001, is a powerful technique to contour the abdomen and flanks. It has not gained widespread use as concerns exist about increased complications related to wound healing and thromboembolism.

Objectives.—The authors review the existing literature on lipoabdominoplasty and discuss their experiences with the technique in a retrospective case series.

Methods.—A literature search of PubMed/MEDLINE using the search terms *lipoabdominoplasty and abdominoplasty* was performed by 2 independent investigators. The charts of 85 consecutive patients who underwent lipoabdominoplasty between February 2007 and July 2012 were reviewed.

Results.—A combined 1316 lipoabdominoplasty patients had results reported in the literature. Of these patients, 21 of 1316 (1.6%) developed seroma, 5 of 1032 (0.5%) experienced hematoma, 6 of 1032 (0.6%) experienced venous thromboembolism, and 3 of 1032 (0.3%) developed pulmonary embolism. In our case series, all patients were women with an average age of 48 years (range, 27-70 years), average body mass index of 25.2 (17.7-35.5), average follow-up of 8 months (range, 1-54 months), average lipoaspirate of 1605 mL (range, 150-5350 mL), and average weight of resected tissue of 1039 g (range, 128-4838 g). The average operative time was 225 minutes (range, 88-435 minutes), and average time in recovery prior to discharge was 124 minutes (range, 33-270 minutes). Seroma occurred in 20 of 85 patients, 1 patient developed deep venous thrombosis (DVT), 1 patient developed cellulitis, and 1 patient developed an abscess.

Conclusion.—Lipoabdominoplasty is a safe and effective procedure in appropriately selected patients. Performing the procedure in an outpatient setting requires attention to multiple factors in the perioperative period to ensure safe patient outcomes. Larger prospective studies should be performed to evaluate best practices regarding rare complications such as DVT or pulmonary embolism.

▶ The literature review portion of this paper confirms that lipoabdominoplasty (including liposuction of the abdominal flap with minimal lateral undermining) is safe, and publications by other authors show its effectiveness in improving abdominal contour. The details of this technique are in the report by Saldanha et al.[1] As for the author's personal series, there was a very high incidence of seromas, and they intend to use progressive tension sutures to address this problem.

K. A. Gutowski, MD

Reference

1. Saldanha OR, Pinto EB, Matos WN Jr, Lucon RL, Magalhães F, Bello EM. Lipoabdominoplasty without undermining. *Aesthet Surg J*. 2001;21:518-526.

Use of Abdominal Field Block Injections With Liposomal Bupivicaine to Control Postoperative Pain After Abdominoplasty

Morales R Jr, Mentz H III, Newall G, et al (Plastic Surgeons in Private Practice in Houston, TX; et al)

Aesthet Surg J 33:1148-1153, 2013

Background.—It is well known that improving postoperative pain control in plastic surgery procedures leads to earlier mobilization, shortened hospital stay, reduced hospital costs, and increased patient satisfaction.

Objective.—The authors evaluate the use of abdominal field block injections with liposomal bupivicaine (Exparel; Pacira Pharmaceuticals, Inc, San Diego, California) in postoperative pain management in patients undergoing abdominoplasty with rectus plication.

Methods.—Case records from 64 female patients who underwent abdominoplasty with rectus plication were reviewed. We performed a total of 118 abdominoplasties with rectus plication, alone or in combination with other surgical procedures, from August 2012 to December 2012, but 54 patients were excluded from the series due to inadequate follow-up. Patients received liposomal bupivicaine injections in an abdominal field block fashion. Patient age, height, weight, and smoking status were recorded. Delivery of standardized postoperative intramuscular or intravenous injections and oral pain pills was recorded. Postoperative data and questionnaires were used to evaluate clinical efficacy.

Results.—The average number of procedures (including abdominoplasty with rectus plication) per patient was 7. Average patient body mass index was 27 kg/m^2. Average pain scores were 3.5 (postoperative visit 1) and 2.8 (visit 2). The average number of oral pain pills required was 14 at the first postoperative visit and 11.5 at the second postoperative visit. Patients were able to resume normal activity at an average of 6.4 days.

Conclusions.—Our experience with liposomal bupivicaine injections for regional blocks in abdominoplasty with rectus plication indicates that patients experienced reduced postoperative pain, required less postoperative narcotic medication, and resumed both earlier ambulation and normal activity. Further investigation is warranted with more clinical cases to recommend the use of this medication for routine pain management after an abdominoplasty.

▶ Pain control after abdominoplasty affects patient satisfaction, discharge to home, and activity level. Liposomal bupivacaine may provide analgesia for up to 3 days after injection allowing for reduced postoperative narcotic medication use. This study did not offer a comparison of pain scores or narcotic use compared with non–liposomal bupivacaine patients, and given the high cost of liposomal bupivacaine, it is hard to make a cost/benefit analysis. Also, the ideal use of liposomal bupivacaine (field block, tissue infiltration, transversus abdominis plane block) is not yet known. However, with more emphasis on faster patient recovery, liposomal bupivacaine is likely to be used more frequently.

K. A. Gutowski, MD

Maximizing Chemoprophylaxis Against Venous Thromboembolism in Abdominoplasty Patients With the Use of Preoperative Heparin Administration

Campbell W, Pierson J, Cohen-Shohet R, et al (Univ of Florida, Gainesville)
Ann Plast Surg 72:S94-S96, 2014

Background.—Abdominoplasty is one of the highest risk plastic surgery procedures for venous thromboembolism complications (VTE). Current recommendations for VTE prophylaxis are sequential compression devices (SCDs) in the OR and optional use of subcutaneous heparin after surgery. Subcutaneous heparin has been shown to be safe in other surgical groups.

However, the large raw surface areas and dissection involved in abdominoplasty has been a relative contraindication for preoperative chemoprophylaxis. However, the period while the patient is under general anesthesia and immediately following the procedure is likely the highest risk time period for VTEs. The purpose of this study is to determine if preoperative chemoprophylaxis is safe in these patients.

Methods.—All patients undergoing abdominoplasty by the senior author from January 1, 2005 to January 1, 2012 were retrospectively reviewed. All patients whose operation took place between January 1, 2005 and January 18, 2008 were given SCDs before the induction of anesthesia and heparin (unfractionated) 5000 units SQ on call to the OR. All patients whose operation took place between January 19, 2008 and January 1, 2012 received enoxaparin (low molecular weight heparin) 40 mg SQ on call to the OR and then daily for 2 days postoperatively. These groups were evaluated in regards to overall complication rate, incidence of VTE, and bleeding complications.

Results.—A total of 151 patients underwent abdominoplasty during the study period. One hundred one patients received the SCD/heparin protocol and 50 had the enoxaparin protocol. The groups were similar in regard to pre-morbid conditions and risk factors for VTE. There were no VTEs diagnosed in either group. The overall incidence of any complication was similar between the 2 groups (19% vs. 14%, $P = 0.503$) and similar to other published series. The most common complications were seroma, cellulitis, and minor wound dehiscence. The incidence of bleeding complications was similar between the 2 groups (1% vs. 0%, $P = 1.0$).

Conclusions.—The use of preoperative chemoprophylaxis in patients undergoing abdominoplasty can be done without an increase in bleeding complications or overall complication rate. Furthermore, enoxaparin can also be used preoperatively and continued for 2 more days during the period of time of maximum immobility with easy administration for outpatients via use of a prescription home use kit.

▶ The ideal venous thromboembolism complications (VTE) prophylaxis for abdominoplasty has not been determined, in part due to variation in surgical and anesthesia technique, patient selection, and postoperative protocols that vary between surgeons. Although this study was underpowered to determine if this protocol reduced VTE incidence, it does suggest that preoperative unfractionated heparin and a 2-day course of enoxaparin does not contribute to a significant increase in postoperative bleeding or hematoma formation. At this time, the optimal duration of VTE chemoprophylaxis after abdominoplasty is not known, but it may be reasonable to continue it until a patient is fully ambulatory.

K. A. Gutowski, MD

Use of Autologous Fibrin Glue (Platelet-Poor Plasma) in Abdominal Dermolipectomies

Schettino AM, Franco D, Franco T, et al (Federal University of Rio de Janeiro, Brazil; et al)

Aesthetic Plast Surg 36:1296-1301, 2012

Background.—Autologous plasma is endowed with properties that speed up healing, hemostasis, and adhesiveness, in addition to growth factors. Through an established protocol, it was possible to isolate thrombin, as well as the platelet-rich plasma (PRP) and platelet-poor plasma (PPP) fractions. The purpose of this study was to analyze autologous use of thrombin and PPP to foster adhesion between an abdominal dermoadipose flap and the aponeurotic surface in abdominal dermolipectomies.

Methods.—The data from 40 patients who underwent abdominal dermolipectomies were analyzed, with 20 patients using thrombin and autologous PPP (Plasma group) and 20 patients with no intervention (Control group). An attempt was made to assess adhesive power by quantifying the serohematic liquid volume gauged during the postoperative days (POD), and also noting the incidence of seroma. Other variables such as age and body mass index (BMI) were also analyzed.

Results.—The reduction in the aspiration drain debit was statistically relevant only on the first POD in the Plasma group. There was no reduction in the incidence of seroma in these patients. Similarly, age and BMI did not influence these outcomes.

Conclusion.—The PPP fostered adhesion between the abdominal dermoadipose flap and the aponeurotic surface only on the first POD and had no influence whatsoever on the incidence of seroma. There are few reports on the use of PPP for plastic surgery, particularly the autologous type, opening up possibilities for further research projects to expand its use.

Level of Evidence III

This journal requires that authors assign a level of evidence to each article. For a full description of these Evidence-Based Medicine ratings, please refer to the table of contents or the online instructions to authors www.springer.com/00266.

► Various off-the-shelf and autologous tissue adhesives have been marketed and studied for seroma prevention in abdominoplasty. Most products, however, add additional cost to the procedure but fail to show significant decreases in seroma formation. The platelet-poor plasma used in this study, although less costly, also failed to show any effect. Seroma formation is more complex and may be influenced by postoperative compression, patient activity, and surgical techniques. Current data suggest that progressive tension sutures may be the best option for seroma prevention in abdominoplasty.

K. A. Gutowski, MD

Long-Term Ultrasonographic Evaluation of Midline Aponeurotic Plication During Abdominoplasty

de Castro EJP, Radwanski HN, Pitanguy I, et al (Hospital Dr. Dorio Silva/ Cooperativa de Cirurgia Plastica do Espirito Santo, Vitória, Brazil)

Plast Reconstr Surg 132:333-338, 2013

Background.—The purpose of this study was to evaluate the efficiency of the plication of the anterior rectus sheath during abdominoplasty and the anatomical characteristics of patients with recurrence.

Methods.—Thirty-eight patients were selected. Patients had undergone abdominoplasty between 1 and 5 years previously. Patients were divided into two groups: group A, 18 patients who had undergone surgery 5 years previously; and group B, 20 patients who had undergone surgery 1 year before. All patients were submitted to a complete physical examination by the plastic surgeon to evaluate the abdominal wall. In addition, an ultrasound examination was performed by the same radiologist in all patients to evaluate rectus diastasis recurrence at two levels: in the supraumbilical region and in the infraumbilical region. The insertion of the recti muscles in the costal margin was also assessed. Groups were compared using Fisher's exact test and the *t* test. Groups were similar regarding age, body mass index, number of smokers, physical activity, and number of pregnancies.

Results.—There was no recurrence of diastasis in any cases of the group with a follow-up of more than 5 years, whereas in the 1-year follow-up group there were two cases of recurrence of the diastasis. Only one of the patients who had recurrence of rectus diastasis had a clinical complaint.

Conclusions.—Recurrence of rectus diastasis is not directly related to the length of the follow-up. It may occur within the first year after abdominoplasty. Recurrence of diastasis diagnosed by ultrasound is not related to a clinical complaint.

Clinical Question/Level of Evidence.—Therapeutic, III.

▶ Although uncommon, recurrence of an abdominal wall bulge after abdominoplasty is frustrating and difficult to correct. This small study showed a 5% diastasis recurrence, which was not symptomatic. The authors point out that lateral recti muscle insertion may account for these findings and propose a medial repositioning of the recti sheath instead of just a midline plication.

K. A. Gutowski, MD

Concurrent panniculectomy with open ventral hernia repair has added risk versus ventral hernia repair: An analysis of the ACS-NSQIP database

Fischer JP, Tuggle CT, Wes AM, et al (Perelman School of Medicine at the Hosp of the Univ of Pennsylvania, Philadelphia; Yale School of Medicine, New Haven, CT)

J Plast Reconstr Aesthet Surg 67:693-701, 2014

Background.—Recent studies have assessed the risks and benefits of performing concurrent panniculectomy (PAN) in the setting of hernia repair, gynecologic surgery, and oncologic resections with conflicting results. The aim of this study is to assess the added risk of ventral hernia repair and panniculectomy (VHR-PAN) using the American College of Surgeons National Surgical Quality Improvement Program (ACS-NSQIP) data sets.

Methods.—The 2005–2011 ACS-NSQIP databases were queried to identify all patients undergoing VHR alone or VHR-PAN. Propensity scores were used to account for potential selection bias given the non-randomized assignment of concurrent panniculectomy and the retrospective nature of this study. Multivariate logistic regression analyses were used to assess the impact of concurrent PAN on complications.

Results.—A total of 55,537 patients were identified. Propensity matching yielded two groups of patients: VHR ($n = 1250$) and VHR-PAN ($n = 1250$). Few statistically significant differences existed between matched cohorts. Overall, wound complications ($P < 0.001$), venous thromboembolism ($P = 0.044$), incidence of reoperation ($P < 0.001$), and medical morbidity ($P < 0.001$) were significantly higher in the VHR-PAN group. In an adjusted, fixed-effects analysis, concurrent panniculectomy was associated with wound healing complications (OR = 1.69, $P < 0.001$), increased incidence of unplanned reoperations (OR = 2.08, $P \leq 0.001$), venous thromboembolism (OR = 2.48, $P = 0.043$), and overall medical morbidity (OR = 2.08, $P < 0.001$). Sub-group analysis of wound complications demonstrated that superficial surgical site infections occurred significantly more often in concurrent cases ($P = 0.018$).

Conclusions.—This analysis quantifies the added risk of performing a panniculectomy concurrent with ventral hernia repair, demonstrating higher incidence of wound complications (superficial infections), unplanned reoperations, and VTE.

Level of Evidence.—Prognostic/risk category, level II.

▶ The results of this study, based on a large multicenter validated national registry, suggest significantly higher complication rates when panniculectomy is combined with ventral hernia repair. Although there are possible benefits to combining these procedures (better surgical exposure, increased patient satisfaction, elimination of the pannus in 1 surgery), patients and referring general surgeons also need to be aware of the increased risks.

K. A. Gutowski, MD

Panniculectomy and Abdominoplasty in Patients Undergoing Gynecologic Surgery: A Single Center Case Series of 15 Combined Procedures

Wallace SA, Mericli AF, Taylor PT, et al (Univ of Virginia, Charlottesville)

Ann Plast Surg 71:88-92, 2013

The current obesity epidemic poses significant challenges to surgical specialists striving to safely and effectively deliver medical care. In the United States, approximately 33.3% of men and 35.3% of women are classified as obese. Pelvic surgery, especially in patients with gynecological malignancies and those who require complex surgical procedures carries additional risk because of the increased technical difficulty posed by excess abdominal wall tissues and increased difficulty in providing and maintaining exposure of the appropriate pelvic anatomy. Simultaneous panniculectomy or abdominoplasty in selected patients may provide better access and visualization of the surgical field, reduce operative difficulty, and decrease perioperative morbidity. We retrospectively reviewed our experience in 15 patients undergoing panniculectomy or abdominoplasty in conjunction with gynecologic surgery. This review was conducted after approval by the local institutional review board. Complications were analyzed, and 2 (13%) of the 15 patients were found to have major complications. The only statistically significant finding for prediction of a negative outcome was an association of hypertension and advanced age with increased risk of postoperative transfusion ($P < 0.02$).

► Performing a panniculectomy for better surgical access during a gynecologic or pelvic procedure may be appropriate; however, doing an aesthetic abdominoplasty during the same time may not. Although there are studies that support each option, prolonged procedures on patients with comorbidities and malignancies place them at very high risk for serious complications, including deep vein thrombosis and pulmonary embolism. The decision to proceed with combined procedures should be based on the relative advantages and disadvantages and include a frank discussion with the patient on additional risk.

K. A. Gutowski, MD

Abdominoplasty-Related Nerve Injuries: Systematic Review and Treatment Options

Ducic I, Zakaria HM, Felder JM III, et al (Georgetown Univ Hosp, Washington, DC)

Aesthet Surg J 34:284-297, 2014

Background.—Abdominoplasty is a common cosmetic procedure; nerve injury is an underexplored risk of the procedure.

Objective.—The authors review existing literature to examine the incidence and treatment of nerve injuries after abdominoplasty procedures and provide a treatment algorithm based on their results.

Methods.—A search of the literature on MEDLINE, EMBASE, and the Cochrane Database of Systematic Reviews was undertaken. After full-text review, 23 articles met our criteria. Any mentions of nerve injury, including references to a lack of nerve injury, were documented. All data were pooled for analysis. From our combined data, we calculated the risks of postabdominoplasty nerve injury by dividing the total number of nerve injuries by the total number of patients.

Results.—Pooled data showed that 1.94% of patients sustained specific nerve injury, and 1.02% of patients sustained permanent injury after abdominoplasty. In addition, 7.67% experienced decreased sensation, 1.07% reported chronic pain, and 0.44% reported temporary weakness or paralysis. Nerves directly injured were the lateral femoral cutaneous (1.36% of patients) and iliohypogastric (0.10%) nerves. Nerves injured from surgical positioning were the brachial plexus (0.10%), musculocutaneous (0.10%), radial (0.05%), sciatic (0.19%), and common peroneal (0.05%) nerves.

Conclusions.—Although our results showed a low incidence of postabdominoplasty nerve injury, the lasting impact on affected patients quality of life can be significant. Appropriate and timely treatment by a multidisciplinary team is critical to optimize patient outcomes. Better reporting of nerve injuries in future studies of abdominoplasty will provide more accurate information about the incidence and consequences of these injuries.

Level of Evidence.—4.

► Peripheral nerve injuries after abdominoplasty may be more common than reported, as many patients learn to live with the associated pain or discomfort without having treatment. This report underscores the importance of knowing the anatomic location of the lateral femoral cutaneous nerve and iliohypogastric nerve and avoiding injury during abdominal procedures. Also, the treatment algorithm for suspected nerve injuries should be kept in mind when patients complain of persistent pain after an abdominoplasty.

K. A. Gutowski, MD

Breast Asymmetry and Pectus Excavatum Improvement With Fat Grafting

Quoc CH, Delaporte T, Meruta A, et al (Centre Régional Léon Bérard, Lyon, France)

Aesthet Surg J 33:822-829, 2013

Background.—In women, pectus excavatum malformation can cause modified breast morphology, resulting in mammary asymmetry, which can be increased by placing mammary implants alone. Fat transfer can be an elegant solution to increase the volume and projection of the breast.

Objectives.—The authors discuss their experience treating pectus excavatum with fat transfer (lipomodeling) since 2000.

Methods.—The charts of 19 consecutive patients with a pectus excavatum breast asymmetry who underwent lipomodeling treatment at the authors' facility between January 2000 and November 2011 were retrospectively reviewed. Patients were separated using the Chin classification (type 1, 2, and 3). Data points for each patient included age and body mass index, number of interventions and volume of fat injected during each session, total volume transferred, and postoperative complications. The clinical result was evaluated by the patient and the surgical team on a 4-point scale: very good, good, fair, or poor.

Results.—Most (74%) patients in this series had type 3 Chin pectus excavatum. The average age was 28 years, and the average body mass index was 20.3. The average number of lipomodeling sessions was 1.63, and the average volume of fat transferred was 230 mL per session and 375 mL total. The patients and the surgical team were very satisfied or satisfied in 95% of cases and considered the result fair in 5% of cases. There were no complications.

Conclusions.—Fat transfer for treatment of pectus excavatum yields very good (natural and stable) results and high patient satisfaction rates, which makes this technique our preferred method for treating thoracomammary malformations in pectus excavatum.

▶ Pectus excavatum is a common thoracic deformity that can cause breast asymmetry in women. It can be challenging to correct with breast implants alone because of chest wall irregularities, which cause implant displacement. Aside from more invasive chest wall procedures, which reposition the sternum and ribs, custom made implants are used for aesthetic improvement of the deformity. The authors present acceptable results using fat grafting to improve the deformity, along with the use of breast implants to enhance the chest.

K. A. Gutowski, MD

Breast Asymmetry and Pectus Excavatum Improvement With Fat Grafting

Ho Quoc C, Delaporte T, Meruta A, et al (Centre Régional Léon Bérard, Lyon, France)

Aesthet Surg J 33:822-829, 2013

Background.—In women, pectus excavatum malformation can cause modified breast morphology, resulting in mammary asymmetry, which can be increased by placing mammary implants alone. Fat transfer can be an elegant solution to increase the volume and projection of the breast.

Objectives.—The authors discuss their experience treating pectus excavatum with fat transfer (lipomodeling) since 2000.

Methods.—The charts of 19 consecutive patients with a pectus excavatum breast asymmetry who underwent lipomodeling treatment at the authors' facility between January 2000 and November 2011 were retrospectively reviewed. Patients were separated using the Chin classification (type 1, 2, and 3). Data points for each patient included age and body mass index, number of interventions and volume of fat injected during each session, total volume transferred, and postoperative complications. The clinical result was evaluated by the patient and the surgical team on a 4-point scale: very good, good, fair, or poor.

Results.—Most (74%) patients in this series had type 3 Chin pectus excavatum. The average age was 28 years, and the average body mass index was 20.3. The average number of lipomodeling sessions was 1.63, and the average volume of fat transferred was 230 mL per session and 375 mL total. The patients and the surgical team were very satisfied or satisfied in 95% of cases and considered the result fair in 5% of cases. There were no complications.

Conclusions.—Fat transfer for treatment of pectus excavatum yields very good (natural and stable) results and high patient satisfaction rates, which makes this technique our preferred method for treating thoraco-mammary malformations in pectus excavatum.

▶ Moderate to severe pectus excavatum in women typically results in breast asymmetry that cannot be overcome with breast implants (which in many cases can make the deformity appear worse). Although fat injections do not treat the underlying chest wall deformity, they do allow for more precise addition of volume and breast contouring to the chest deficiency compared with custom implants. Not surprisingly, 2 to 3 treatment sessions were needed to achieve good results. When combined with appropriately sized breast implants, fat grafting can allow for an improved chest wall and breast appearance.

K. A. Gutowski, MD

Posterior Wedge Resection: A More Aesthetic Labiaplasty

Kelishadi SS, Elston JB, Rao AJ, et al (Univ of Louisville, KY)
Aesthet Surg J 33:847-853, 2013

Background.—Hypertrophy of the labia minora is of concern to a subset of adolescents and adult women. The posterior wedge resection is a new labiaplasty technique with an anatomic approach to yield the optimal aesthetic outcome and yet continue the functional achievement of prior techniques.

Objective.—The authors describe the results of their posterior wedge resection technique in a retrospective series of patients.

Methods.—A retrospective chart review was performed of 22 consecutive patients who underwent posterior wedge resection labiaplasty between February 2009 and February 2012. Complications and aesthetic outcomes were reviewed.

Results.—The average age of the patients in this study was 35 years (median, 33 years). Follow-up ranged from 2 weeks to 1.5 years. Two minor complications occurred without further sequelae. At follow-up, none of the patients reported any paresthesias, pain, or problems with penetrating vaginal intercourse.

Conclusions.—An increasing number of labiaplasties are being performed for aesthetic and functional concerns. The posterior wedge resection enables the surgeon to perform labiaplasty easily, safely, and effectively, ensuring symmetry and maintenance of the natural pigment, color, and texture of the defining free edge of the labia minora.

▶ Various labia minora reduction techniques are available to reduce labial hypertrophy, ranging from simple edge excision (which has fewer healing problems but eliminates the normal pigmented labial edge) to complex multiwedge excisions (which may preserve the labial edge but tend to have more healing problems). This posterior edge technique is a modification of other inferior techniques and appears to be easier to design than more complex wedge excisions and yet produces a good aesthetic result.

K. A. Gutowski, MD

Aesthetic Shoulder Augmentation with Silicone Implants

Chung YJ, Jang H (Eve Plastic Surgery Clinic, Seoul, South Korea; Dopo Branch of Yeongam Public Health Ctr, South Korea)

Aesthetic Plast Surg 38:41-48, 2014

Background.—Men with narrower shoulders may appear less muscular than other men. Deltoid muscle underdevelopment or atrophy, a condition commonly linked to narrow shoulder issues, may be associated with congenital deformity, trauma, or neoplasm. For some people, regular exercise does not effectively develop the deltoid muscle region. Some people naturally have a smaller build than others. Even with developed deltoid muscles, these people still appear to be small. The authors have performed lateral shoulder augmentation with silicone implants for 4 years. Based on their experience, this procedure stands as a reliable solution for men with narrow shoulders.

Methods.—Lateral shoulder augmentation with silicone implants was developed and used for 81 patients between April 2009 and April 2013. None of the patients had shoulder deformities except for two patients (one patient with Poland's syndrome and one patient with Sprengel's deformity). The implants were placed through a horizontal axillary crease incision in a plane dissected between the deltoid fascia and muscle.

Results.—All augmentation or correction procedures have been met with complete patient approval. Five patients had minor complications such as hematoma and implement displacement. However, all these complications were resolved to the satisfaction of the patients.

Conclusion.—When silicone implants are used to achieve purely aesthetic improvements, successful shoulder augmentation procedures are observed.

Level of Evidence IV.—This journal requires that authors assign a level of evidence to each submission to which Evidence-Based Medicine rankings are applicable. This excludes Review Articles, Book Reviews, and manuscripts that concern Basic Science, Animal Studies, Cadaver Studies, and Experimental Studies. For a full description of these Evidence-Based Medicine ratings, please refer to the Table of Contents or the online Instructions to Authors http://www.springer.com/00266.

▶ Common implants for body contouring include breast, pectoral, calf, and gluteal. Less common are biceps, triceps, and abdominal implants. This report describes a large series of soft silicone implants designed for shoulder augmentation placed using local anesthesia and sedation. Complications were low and results were reasonable. Although it is too early to see if this new implant catches on, it may be considered in cases of deltoid hypoplasia.

K. A. Gutowski, MD

Is the High Superior Tension Technique an Equivalent Substitute for Progressive Tension Sutures in Postbariatric Abdominoplasty? A Comparison Prospective Study

Margara A, Boriani F, Granchi D, et al (Rizzoli Inst and Univ of Bologna, Italy)
Plast Reconstr Surg 133:544-549, 2014

Background.—The addition of progressive tension sutures to the abdominoplasty technique is advocated to reduce the risk of several complications. High superior tension abdominoplasty is another technique aimed at reducing tension at the prepubic suture line and improving cosmesis of the umbilical area.

Methods.—A cohort of massive weight loss patients undergoing abdominoplasty, treated with the progressive tension suture technique in association with the high superior tension technique (group A), was followed up and compared to a cohort of patients who underwent high superior tension abdominoplasty (group B). Several variables including rate of complications and patient satisfaction were explored to determine any possible benefit deriving from the combination of progressive tension suture and high superior tension techniques in the abdominoplasty.

Results.—A total of 90 patients were included in the study, of whom 34 were in group A and 56 were in group B. No statistically significant difference was found between the two groups in terms of duration of the procedure, hospitalization time, rate of complications, drained volume, and patient or physician satisfaction.

Conclusion.—No beneficial effect appears to derive from the progressive tension suture technique in massive weight loss patients undergoing abdominoplasty, provided that the high superior tension technique is performed as an adjunct to the traditional method.

▶ Progressive tension sutures (PTS) are more accepted in abdominoplasty as an alternative to using subcutaneous drains. Unfortunately, in this study, drains were used in both patient groups, so the conclusion that the PTS are not beneficial is not valid.

K. A. Gutowski, MD

Liposuction, Fat Transfer, and Tissue Fillers

Comparison of Limited-Undermining Lipoabdominoplasty and Traditional Abdominoplasty Using Laser Fluorescence Imaging

Roostaeian J, Harris R, Farkas JP, et al (Univ of California, Los Angeles; Univ of Texas Southwestern, Dallas; Plastic Surgeon in Private Practice in Paramus, NJ)

Aesthet Surg J 34:741-747, 2014

Background.—Body contouring that involves abdominoplasty and/or liposuction is a common cosmetic surgery procedure. Although single-staged lipoabdominoplasty has gained popularity, safety concerns remain.

Objectives.—The authors compared abdominal flap perfusion and overall complication rates for traditional abdominoplasty and limited-undermining lipoabdominoplasty.

Methods.—Eighteen abdominoplasty patients were evaluated in a prospective study. All patients were nonsmokers and lacked major comorbidities. The control group ($n = 9$) underwent traditional abdominoplasty with wide undermining. The study group ($n = 9$) underwent abdominoplasty with limited undermining as well as liposuction of the abdominal flap. The groups were similar with respect to age and body mass index. Patients received follow-up for an average of 97 days. Fluorescence imaging was utilized for perfusion studies. Results and complications were documented, and statistical significance was ascertained via the Student *t* test.

Results.—Neither group had major complications or revisions. Minor complications included an exposed suture, resulting in delayed wound healing, in the control group. A patient in the study group had a small area of fat necrosis and a small seroma, neither of which required further treatment. No significant difference in abdominal flap perfusion was found between the control (57%) and study (50%) groups based on fluorescence levels relative to a designated baseline reference marker.

Conclusions.—Results of the study indicate that no significant differences exist between the 2 operations with respect to the rates of abdominal flap perfusion or complications.

Level of Evidence.—3.

► This may be the first study to demonstrate similar abdominal flap tissue perfusion between traditional abdominoplasty and limited-undermining lipoabdominoplasty (LUL). Although LUL is becoming more accepted, many surgeons still have concerns about performing extensive liposuction of an abdominoplasty flap because of possible flap vascular compromise. These findings add to the already published clinical evidence that a properly done LUL does not have a higher risk of complications.[1,2]

K. A. Gutowski, MD

References

1. Saldanha OR, De Souza Pinto EB, Mattos WN Jr, et al. Lipoabdominoplasty with selective and safe undermining. *Aesthetic Plast Surg*. 2003;27:322-327.
2. Saldanha OR, Federico R, Daher PF, et al. Lipoabdominoplasty. *Plast Reconstr Surg*. 2009;124:934-942.

The Effectiveness and Safety of Combining Laser-Assisted Liposuction and Abdominoplasty

Aboelatta YA, Abdelaal MM, Bersy NA (Ain Shams Univ, Abbassia, Cairo, Egypt)

Aesthetic Plast Surg 38:49-56, 2014

Background.—Lipoabdominoplasty is nearly a daily aesthetic procedure. Despite the emergence of laser-assisted liposuction, to date, it has not been clearly evaluated combined with abdominoplasty. This prospective study aimed to evaluate the effectiveness and safety of laser-assisted liposuction relative to traditional liposuction combined with high-lateral-tension abdominoplasty.

Methods.—This study investigated 36 consecutive female patients who underwent high-lateral-tension abdominoplasty combined with liposuction of the upper central abdomen and both flanks. The patients were divided into three equal groups based on the technique used for liposuction. Group 1 underwent conventional liposuction with abdominoplasty. Group 2 underwent a mixture of conventional and laser-assisted liposuction with abdominoplasty. Group 3 underwent laser-assisted liposuction with abdominoplasty.

Results.—The patients in groups 2 and 3 had a better aesthetic outcome than those in group 1 with regard to abdominal contour and skin tightness. No major complications were observed in groups 1 and 2. The patients in group 3 had a higher incidence of complications (3 seromas, 3 central necroses and dehiscence), and one patient underwent secondary sutures.

Conclusion.—Laser-assisted liposuction combined with abdominoplasty in the lateral abdomen seems to be a safe technique with good aesthetic outcomes. Although the combined use of laser-assisted liposuction in the lateral and central abdomen can achieve relatively better aesthetic results, it is associated with significant complications, and its use cannot be supported. Proper laser parameters in the central abdominal area still need further study.

Level of Evidence IV.—This journal requires that authors assign a level of evidence to each article. For a full description of these Evidence-Based Medicine ratings, please refer to the Table of Contents or the online Instructions to Authors www.springer.com/00266.

▶ It is rare to find a report that is critical of a new liposuction technology. The authors found that central abdominal flap laser-assisted liposuction was associated with more seromas, central necrosis, and dehiscence compared with traditional liposuction. As with all energy devices, the purported benefits need to be weighed against the real risks.

K. A. Gutowski, MD

Nonexcisional Tissue Tightening: Creating Skin Surface Area Reduction During Abdominal Liposuction by Adding Radiofrequency Heating

Duncan DI (Plastic Surgeon in Private Practice in Fort Collins, CO)

Aesthet Surg J 33:1154-1166, 2013

Background.—Recent publications show that heat-mediated tissue tightening is a promising treatment for the lax abdomen and may provide better long-term outcomes than traditional suction-assisted liposuction (SAL).

Objectives.—The author evaluates the degree and duration of skin surface area contraction, as well as the influence of anatomic location of the treatment region on the degree of tissue tightening, in a study comparing SAL alone vs SAL plus radiofrequency-assisted liposuction (RFAL).

Methods.—In this prospective, randomized, split abdominal study, 12 consecutive patients were treated with SAL alone on 1 side and with SAL plus RFAL on the other side. Each patient had 4 (3 × 3-cm) squares—2 per treatment type—tattooed in the lower abdominal region (2 on the right and 2 on the left). The surface area of these squares was measured with the Vectra computerized measurement system (Canfield, Inc, Fairfield, New Jersey) at pretreatment, at 6 weeks posttreatment, and at 1 year posttreatment. All measurements were subjected to statistical analysis using predictive analytic software and were evaluated for statistical significance.

Results.—In regions treated with SAL alone, there was a 10.4% mean skin surface area contraction at 6 weeks and 8.3% at 1 year posttreatment. The mean skin surface area reduction was 25.8% in regions treated with radiofrequency plus SAL at 6 weeks and at 1 year. The anatomic location of each square (medial vs lateral) did not statistically correlate with more or less tissue tightening.

Conclusions.—Radiofrequency-assisted tissue tightening, when applied in conjunction with SAL, is effective in achieving greater skin surface area reduction.

▶ This may be the first published report to objectively show that skin tightening after liposuction combined with internal radiofrequency (RF) is significantly better than liposuction alone. The clinical photographs also confirm a difference in skin tightening between the RF treated and non-treated side. The RF device used (BodyTite by Invasix) is not approved by the US Food and Drug Administration as of early 2014, but it may be worthwhile to follow this technology as it goes through the regulatory approval process.

K. A. Gutowski, MD

Analgesic Efficacy of Lidocaine for Suction-Assisted Lipectomy with Tumescent Technique under General Anesthesia: A Randomized, Double-Masked, Controlled Trial

Danilla S, Fontbona M, de Valdés VD, et al (Hospital Clínico J. J. Aguirre, Santiago, Chile; Clínica Alemana, Santiago, Chile; Hospital Militar de Santiago, Chile; et al)

Plast Reconstr Surg 132:327-332, 2013

Background.—Suction-assisted lipectomy is one of the most common procedures performed in plastic surgery. To minimize blood loss and to obtain adequate analgesia, a liquid solution is infiltrated into the subcutaneous plane before suction. The objective of this study was to determine whether the use of lidocaine in the infiltration solution reduces postoperative pain.

Methods.—A prospective, randomized, double-masked, clinical trial was designed. Each side of patients' body zones to be treated with suction-assisted lipectomy was randomized to receive infiltration solution with or without lidocaine. Treatment allocation was performed using computer-generated random numbers in permuted blocks of eight. Pain was assessed using the visual analogue scale and registered 1, 6, 12, 18, and 24 hours after the procedure.

Results.—The trial was stopped after a first interim analysis. The use of lidocaine in the dilute solution reduced pain by 0.5 point on the visual analogue scale (95 percent CI, 0.3 to 0.8; $p < 0.001$). The effect was independent of the suctioned body zone ($p = 0.756$), and lasted until 18 hours after surgery. Its analgesic effect was lost at the 24-hour postoperative control. Pain increased an average of 0.018 point on the visual analogue scale per hour (95 percent CI, 0.001 to 0.036; $p = 0.043$).

Conclusions.—The use of lidocaine in the infiltration solution is effective in postoperative pain control until 18 hours after surgery. Nevertheless, its clinical effect is limited and clinically irrelevant, and therefore it is no longer used by the authors.

Clinical Question/Level of Evidence.—Therapeutic, I.

▶ This study suggests that the addition of lidocaine to infiltration fluid before liposuction is not necessary for pain control, as the analgesic effect is only a 0.5-point improvement on a 10-point scale. Although the study was well designed (each patient had half of their body infiltrated with lidocaine-containing solution and the other half did not receive lidocaine), it did not account for the possibility that the lidocaine infiltrated on one side was distributed by the blood stream to the opposite side. Because intravenous lidocaine injection has been found to reduce postoperative pain, and because blood lidocaine levels increase after subcutaneous infiltration, it is possible that the entire body benefited from lidocaine use on only one side. For this reason, these findings may not give us a definitive answer regarding the use of lidocaine in liposuction. Also, these findings only apply to liposuction done under general anesthesia. When done under sedation anesthesia, some type of tissue level pain control is still needed for patient comfort during liposuction.

K. A. Gutowski, MD

Suction-assisted lipectomy fails to improve cardiovascular metabolic markers of disease: A meta-analysis

Danilla S, Longton C, Valenzuela K, et al (Hospital Clínico Universidad de Chile, Santiago; Pontificia Universidad Católica de Chile, Santiago; Universidad de Chile, Santiago; et al)

J Plast Reconstr Aesthetic Surg 66:1557-1563, 2013

Background.—The purpose of this study was to determine whether suction-assisted lipectomy (SAL) decreases the incidence of early cardiovascular disease risk factors or its biochemical and clinical risk indicators.

Methods.—A systematic review of the literature was performed by conducting a predefined, sensitive search in MEDLINE without limiting the year of publication or language. The extracted data included the basal characteristics of the patients, the surgical technique, the amount of fat extracted, the cardiovascular risk factors and the biochemical and clinical markers monitored over time. The data were analysed using pooled curves, risk ratios and standardised means with meta-analytical techniques.

Results.—Fifteen studies were identified involving 357 patients. In all of the studies, measurements of predefined variables were recorded before and after the SAL procedure. The median follow-up was 3 months (interquartile range (IQR) 1–6, range 0.5–10.5). The mean amount of extracted fat ranged from 2063 to 16,300 ml, with a mean ± standard deviation (SD) of 6138 ± 4735 ml. After adjusting for time and body mass index (BMI), leptin and fasting insulin were the only markers that were significantly associated with the amount of aspirated fat. No associations were observed for high sensitive C-reactive protein (hCRP), interleukin-6 (IL-6), adiponectin, resistin, tumour necrosis factor-α (TNF-α), Homeostasis Model of Assessment (HOMA), total cholesterol, high-density lipoprotein (HDL), low-density lipoprotein (LDL), triglycerides, free fatty acids or systolic blood pressure.

Conclusions.—Based on the results of our analysis, we conclude that there is no evidence to support the hypothesis that subcutaneous fat removal reduces early cardiovascular or metabolic disease, its markers or its risk factors.

▶ A few studies that demonstrated favorable changes in metabolic markers after liposuction were able to generate media coverage. However, this meta-analysis of 15 studies did not see any improvements. Until large prospective trials are done, claims of liposuction offering cardiovascular health benefits should not be made.

K. A. Gutowski, MD

A New Osmidrosis Procedure, the Scrape and Suction Technique: Review of 4,322 Patients

Kim H-G (Seoul Plastic Surgery Ctr, South Korea)

Aesthetic Plast Surg 38:282-287, 2014

Background.—Axillary osmidrosis causes unpleasant odors and profuse sweating, resulting in social and psychological problems. Many treatment modalities have been attempted and liposuction is preferred because of the minimal scar, although the problem of a high recurrence rate still exists. The aim of this study was to introduce and evaluate the efficacy of a new technique to treat axillary osmidrosis using a liposuction machine.

Methods.—From January 2002 to December 2012, a total of 4,322 patients with axillary osmidrosis were treated with a new technique that combines suction with aggressive scraping. Treatment outcomes were assessed by a patient survey in the outpatient clinic at least 6 months after surgery. Permanent tissue biopsies were obtained from the left axilla before surgery and from the right axilla after surgery and compared to each other.

Results.—Ninety-five percent of the patients ($n = 4{,}092$) were very satisfied with the result, including the postoperative scars, and responded that they never or hardly ever experienced symptoms of axillary osmidrosis postoperatively. Recurrences occurred in 230 patients (5%) and most resolved after additional procedures, except 36 cases (0.8%). The tissue biopsy showed complete excision of the apocrine glands and a well-cut cross-sectional view of the dermis. Superficial epidermal necrosis occurred in 41 patients, probably due to hematoma, and 32 patients of the 41 (78.0%) were treated successfully without any revisional procedures.

Conclusion.—The new technique of scraping and suctioning with a newly designed liposuction machine achieved minimal scars, low recurrence rates, and very high patient satisfaction. This technique can be a simple and effective treatment modality for the treatment of axillary osmidrosis.

Level of Evidence IV.—This journal requires that authors assign a level of evidence to each article. For a full description of these Evidence-Based Medicine ratings, please refer to the Table of Contents or the online Instructions to Authors www.springer.com/00266.

▶ Medical treatment of axillary hyperhidrosis includes neuromodulator injections and more recently external microwave application (midaDri), as well as direct gland removal using a liposuction technique. However, the suction technique frequently does not completely remove all apocrine tissue, and recurrence is common. The difference in this report is the use of a modified traditional liposuction cannula so that 2 apertures, 2 mm apart, acted as knives and aspirated the sweat glands more efficiently—not only in the subcutaneous tissue but also in the dermal layers. Because the dermal tissue is also treated from the deep surface, a few cases (1%) of skin necrosis occurred and required small skin grafts. Although the results are favorable, the average follow-up was only 9 months.

K. A. Gutowski, MD

Scar Asymmetry After Abdominoplasty: The Unexpected Role of Seroma

di Summa PG, Wettstein R, Erba P, et al (Univ Hosp of Lausanne, Switzerland)

Ann Plast Surg 71:461-463, 2013

Achievement of symmetry remains one of the goals of cosmetic procedures. Interestingly, scar asymmetry after abdominoplasty has been rarely considered a complication. However, this can have a significant impact on patient and surgeon satisfaction. This study identifies silent seromas as a potential cause of scar asymmetry.

Among abdominoplasty procedures in a university hospital institution over a 30 months' period (October 1, 2007 to April 1, 2010), we retrospectively identified 6 patients who developed abdominal scar asymmetry only 3 months postoperatively and without any early warning complications (hematoma, seroma, or infection). Clinical examination was completed by abdominal diagnostic ultrasonography. Seroma capsulectomy under local anesthesia was performed in all cases.

In all patients clinically presenting late abdominal scar asymmetry, ultrasonography confirmed the presence of an encapsulated chronic seroma. Surgical capsulectomy under local anesthesia resulted in reestablishment of former symmetry and high patient satisfaction. No complications such as wound infection, dehiscence, hematoma, or recurrence of seroma were detected after revision surgery.

In our experience, fibrous capsule due to chronic seromas resulted in abdominal scar deviation and asymmetry. Surgical capsulectomy followed by wearing of compressive garments resulted to be an effective treatment with pleasant aesthetic outcome and no seroma recurrence. Silent seromas should be considered as a possible etiologic factor of scar asymmetries appearing during late follow-up after abdominoplasty.

▶ Small seromas may go unnoticed, but as this report reminds us, they may also compromise results. In this series, seromas ranging in volume from 70 to 160 cc were small enough not to be seen as a bulge but were large enough to cause downward scar curvature. Surgeons should keep this in mind when assessing abdominoplasty scars.

K. A. Gutowski, MD

6 Breast

General

Tuberous Breast Correction by Fat Grafting

Delay E, Sinna R, Ho Quoc C (Centre Régional Léon Bérard, Lyon, France)

Aesthet Surg J 33:522-528, 2013

Introduction.—Tuberous breast is a rare malformation that has negative physical and psychological impacts during puberty. A range of surgical techniques has been used to correct breast shape and volume in this context, including a combination of skin plasty and mammary gland remodeling, as well as prostheses and locoregional flaps. The authors have used fat grafting as a complementary technique to correct tuberous breasts since 1998.

Objectives.—The authors discuss application of their lipomodeling technique for correction of tuberous breast deformity.

Methods.—The charts of tuberous breast patients treated consecutively over an 11-year period (n = 31) solely with fat grafting (ie, without using an implant) were retrospectively reviewed. Each breast deformation was graded according to the Grolleau classification. The number of sessions and the mean transfer of fat volume by lipomodeling session were recorded. Patient and surgeon satisfaction were evaluated.

Results.—Of the 31 patients in this series, 18 had bilateral formations and 13 had unilateral malformations. The mean patient age was 23 years, and the mean body mass index was 21.9. A single session (mean transfer volume, 158 mL; range, 90-253 mL) was required in 14 (45%) cases. A second session (mean transfer volume, 226 mL; range, 100-316 mL) was necessary in the remaining 55% of cases. Mean follow-up period after the last fat transfer session was 6.5 years (range, 1.5-11 years). Patients were very satisfied in 94% of cases (n = 29) and satisfied in 6% (n = 2). The surgical team rated 94% of cases as being successful or very successful. No complications were observed. One patient developed hypertrophy of the treated breast following weight gain and thus required breast reduction. Imaging performed preoperatively and 1 year postoperatively did not reveal any anomalies other than oil cysts.

Conclusion.—Fat grafting is a reliable technique that produces excellent results and high levels of patient satisfaction for the treatment of tuberous

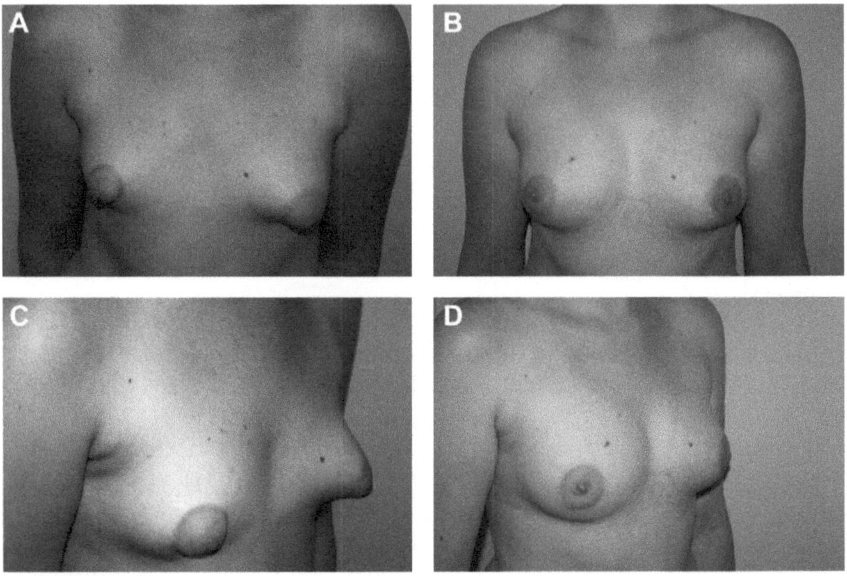

FIGURE 3.—(A, C, E) This 18-year-old woman presented with bilateral tuberous breasts (Grolleau type 3). (B, D, F) One year after 2 sessions of bilateral lipomodeling (116 and 190 mL in the right breast; 80 and then 110 mL in the left breast). (Reprinted from Delay E, Sinna R, Ho Quoc C. Tuberous breast correction by fat grafting. *Aesthet Surg J*. 2013;33:522-528, Copyright 2013, with permission from The American Society for Aesthetic Plastic Surgery, Inc.)

breast. The aesthetic outcome is natural, implant free, and long lasting (Fig 3).

▶ These authors present rather remarkable results, and quite frankly they are almost astonishing and among the best I have seen, especially considering that most of their patients were Grolleau type 2 and 3. I am at a loss to explain how you can release fibrous bands using a trochar or cannula without any visualization. Even more spectacular is how they were able to increase the small base circumference of these constricted breasts using only a cannula or trochar? The authors also seem to have addressed the herniated areola in some fashion in the patient shown in Fig 3, but it is unclear how this occurred with the technique described. It is interesting that these authors do not seem to agree with the prevailing notion in US plastic surgical circles that external breast expansion and fat grafting the (BRAVA-AFT) system is preferred in these breasts.[1] Of course, the caveat espoused at the beginning of the article—"this technique has a learning curve and requires precise technique"—should be taken to heart by those who have not seen this surgery performed by someone with a great deal of experience. Much more research is required to document the efficacy and long-term benefits of the use of fat grafting in these difficult breast reconstructions and whether such grafting is facilitated by external expansion of the breast.

S. H. Miller, MD

Reference

1. Khouri R, Del Vecchio D. Breast reconstruction and augmentation using pre-expansion and autologous fat transplantation. *Clin Plast Surg*. 2009;36:269-280.

Mastopexy and Reduction

The Impact of Body Mass Index on Reduction Mammaplasty: A Multicenter Analysis of 2492 Patients

Gust MJ, Smetona JT, Persing JS, et al (Northwestern Univ, Chicago, IL; Loyola Univ Stritch School of Medicine, Chicago, IL)

Aesthet Surg J 33:1140-1147, 2013

Background.—Reduction mammaplasty is commonly performed in women who are considered obese by the body mass index (BMI) classification of the World Health Organization.

Objectives.—The authors compare complication rates among breast reduction patients, stratified by BMI, across multiple institutions.

Methods.—A retrospective analysis was performed of all reduction mammaplasties in the database of the National Surgical Quality Improvement Program for 2006 through 2010. Demographic, comorbidity, and BMI data were collected. Data on medical and surgical complications, reoperation, and mortality were collected through 30 days postsurgery.

Results.—Of 2492 patients, 55% were considered obese (BMI >30). The overall rate of surgical complications was 4.0%, increasing from 2.4% for BMI <25 to 7.1% for BMI >45 ($P = .006$), with an adjusted odds ratio of 2.97 for BMI >45 versus BMI <25. The most common surgical complication was superficial surgical site infection; it was found in 2.9% of patients, increasing from 2.1% for BMI <25 to 5.1% for BMI >45 ($P = .03$). The medical complication rate was 0.6%, and the reoperation rate was 2.1%. There were no deaths. A maximal point analysis showed that BMI ≥39 was associated with a significantly higher complication rate, with an odds ratio of 2.38.

Conclusions.—Reduction mammaplasty is a safe surgical procedure, even when performed on obese patients. However, patients with higher BMI have a greater risk of surgical site complications. This risk should be discussed preoperatively with obese patients.

Level of Evidence.—3.

▶ Breast reduction is considered a safe procedure, but frequently minor incision healing or skin necrosis problems are encountered, which result in delayed healing. As most plastic surgeons have encountered, obese patients tend to have more healing complications after surgery. This study gives strong support regarding a higher surgical site complication rate for breast reduction in obese patients, particularly those with a body mass index greater than 39, and should be used in counseling patients before surgery.

K. A. Gutowski, MD

Augmentation and Silicone

The Ever-Changing Role of Biofilms in Plastic Surgery

Constantine RS, Constantine FC, Rohrich RJ (Univ of Pennsylvania, Philadelphia; Univ of Texas Southwestern Med Ctr, Dallas)

Plast Reconstr Surg 133:865e-872e, 2014

The goal of this article is to present a brief background of biofilms and how they pertain to plastic surgery. Of particular interest are how biofilms affect breast prosthesis and their subsequent complications. The authors also present information on how biofilms are involved in soft-tissue filler complications. After a brief review of the pathophysiology of biofilms and their effect on plastic surgery, the authors propose a revised algorithm to assist in guiding the plastic surgeon when faced with complications that involve biofilms that involves more rapid diagnosis and treatment using polymerase chain reaction technology. This article is a review of recent literature.

▶ Biofilms are implicated in many infections, particularly those associated with medical implants and indwelling devices. Difficulty in diagnosis of biofilm infections is in part due to the specific growth media and culture conditions that are not found in most hospital laboratories. Special techniques such as rapid polymerase chain reaction testing may be needed to make a diagnosis and identify the specific pathogen. In plastic surgery, biofilms should be considered in cases of capsular contracture after implant breast augmentation, late-presenting soft-tissue filler complications, and other inflammatory or infectious problems associated with prosthetic devices.

K. A. Gutowski, MD

A systematic review of the use of Botulinum toxin type A with subpectoral breast implants

Winocour S, Murad MH, Bidgoli-Moghaddam M, et al (Mayo Clinic, Rochester, MN)

J Plast Reconstr Aesthet Surg 67:34-41, 2014

Objective.—To determine the efficacy of Botulinum toxin A (BTX-A) injections for pain relief following placement of subpectoral tissue expanders and breast implants.

Methods.—MEDLINE and EMBASE were searched from their inception to December 2012 to identify studies reporting the efficacy of perioperative BTX-A injections following breast surgery with subpectoral prostheses. Study designs included controlled and uncontrolled studies.

Results.—Seven studies met the inclusion criteria (2 prospective controlled cohort, 3 retrospective cohort and 2 case series). Five studies assessed the efficacy of BTX-A and three measured pain improvement as a primary outcome. The studies enrolled 427 women: 91.8% received intraoperative BTX-A injection at the time of tissue expander breast reconstruction and 4.7% following augmentation mammaplasty. Only 3.5% of women received BTX-A injections in the postoperative setting. Overall, all the studies demonstrated improvement in pain and favorable side effect profile without any major adverse effects. However, the quality of this evidence was low.

Conclusion.—The results of this systematic review suggest that BTX-A may alleviate postoperative pain associated with the placement of subpectoral tissue expanders and implants. The available data on outcome assessment of this practice are inconsistent and lack methodological rigor. With paucity of high-level evidence to support this practice in implant-based breast surgery, further studies are needed.

▶ This is a potentially very interesting therapeutic concept: the use of Botulism toxin type A (BTX-A) to alleviate pain after submuscular placements of breast implants or tissue expanders (TE) during the course of breast reconstruction. One can certainly understand that BTX-A, if injected into one or several of the muscles used in submuscular placement of an implant or TE, could, by virtue of relaxing said muscle(s), reduce pain. Unexpected was not only that effect but also a direct reduction of pain using BTX-A through inhibition of a neurotransmitter, substance P. This is clearly intriguing information, but this study merely shows the very low level of evidence on which to base the use of BTX-A in these settings. Before performing a large multicenter trial, it will be necessary to work out appropriate dose response curves, how many muscles need to be injected, and the routes of administration. It is equally obvious that a rather large, adequately powered prospective, blinded study is needed of the effect of BTX-A on the pain associated with submuscular breast implants and another study to document the benefits associated with tissue expansion breast reconstruction.

S. H. Miller, MD

Use of Porcine Acellular Dermal Matrix in Revisionary Cosmetic Breast Augmentation

Pozner JN, White JB, Newman MI (Cleveland Clinic Florida, Weston; ARC Plastic Surgery, Hollywood, FL)

Aesthet Surg J 33:681-690, 2013

Background.—Aesthetic breast augmentation can be fraught with postoperative complications, particularly capsular contracture (CC), skin surface irregularities, and implant or inframammary fold malposition. Similar complications have been addressed successfully in reconstructive breast surgery with acellular dermal matrix (ADM) products.

Objective.—The authors present their initial experience with porcine ADM (PADM) in aesthetic breast augmentation.

Methods.—Retrospective chart review was performed for 93 consecutive patients (179 breasts) who underwent revisionary cosmetic breast augmentation with or without mastopexy between May 2009 and September 2012. Porcine ADM (Strattice; Lifecell Corp, Branchburg, New Jersey) was placed bilaterally in 74 patients and unilaterally in 19 patients. All patients were operated upon by 1 surgeon (J.N.P.). Product use description and complications were recorded, including infection, extrusion, CC, and implant malposition.

Results.—Average follow-up was 12 months (range, 1-39 months). There were 2 major complications (1.6% of breasts): an infection in 1 breast that required implant explantation approximately 2 weeks postoperatively and an extrusion that required PADM removal. Two additional patients had high-riding implants resulting from folded PADM that required revision; both cases were corrected by excising the folded PADM segment. Seven other patients required office procedures to correct minor imperfections. Two CC recurrences were suspected (1 patient) in the 76 breasts that underwent capsulectomy and PADM placement.

Conclusions.—Porcine ADM demonstrated great utility as an adjunct in revisionary cosmetic breast surgery. The product helped to provide good aesthetic outcomes with low complication rates. Prospective, randomized trials may prove helpful in defining the role of PADM further in these challenging cases.

▶ This series adds more support to the observations that certain acellular dermal matrix (ADM) products may decrease the recurrence of capsular contracture. ADM is also useful for correction of implant malposition, particularly when lateral or inferior (bottoming out). When a capsulorrhaphy is not possible (because of poor tissue quality) or a new pocket cannot be created, ADM should be considered. It is important to discuss this with patients before surgery, as intraoperative findings may dictate the need for ADM use. Likewise, a discussion regarding the additional costs of ADM needs to include the possibility of further revisional surgery if ADM is not used. The risks of increase seroma formation and possible increase in infection must also be considered.

K. A. Gutowski, MD

Experimental total wrapping of breast implants with acellular dermal matrix: A preventive tool against capsular contracture in breast surgery?

Schmitz M, Bertram M, Kneser U, et al (Friedrich Alexander Univ of Erlangen-Nuremberg, Germany)

J Plast Reconstr Aesthet Surg 66:1382-1389, 2013

Background.—Capsular contracture remains a hitherto unsolved complication after implantation of silicone gel-filled breast prostheses. Based on clinical and experimental data, the use of an acellular dermal matrix as a sheath around implants may lead to lesser capsular contracture acting as a proposed biological environment mimicking wound bed tissue. The aim of our study was to analyse the tissue reaction after implantation of silicone prosthesis with and without an envelope of acellular dermal matrix.

Methods.—Implantation of 60 silicone prostheses in the back of Lewis rats were carried out, randomly paired taking one rat from group A and one from group B. Group A included implants completely enveloped with xenogenic acellular dermis and group B undraped silicone implants. At 3, 6 and 12 weeks postoperatively, the samples were explanted and subjected to histological and immunohistochemical evaluation.

Results.—A new myofibroblast tissue layer was identified in proximity to the implant in both groups. The thickness of the layer in group A was continuously thinner than in group B regarding the different explantation time points. Implants completely wrapped with acellular dermal matrix showed significantly lesser inflammatory signs at 3 and 12 weeks after implantation compared to controls. Cell proliferation after 12 weeks was significantly decreased in group A.

Conclusion.—The slight myofibroblast layer and reduced rate of inflammation and proliferation in the treatment group show a positive effect of total acellular dermal matrix envelope and hypothesise the decrease of capsular contracture in long-term periods.

▶ This is an early and preliminary study of the effects of using a single type of xenogenic acellular dermal matrix (Strattice) as a total wrap around animal-sized silicone testicular implant in Lewis rats. The authors note that cell proliferation at 12 weeks was less in the tissues surrounding the totally wrapped silicone implant than in the nonwrapped implant. But several issues remain unclear: (1) A thin collagenous layer was found around both sets of implants regardless of wrapping. (2) The developing myofibroblast layer increased in both groups when examined at 3 and 6 weeks, but was less at 12, although the degree of thickness was by no means stable at this time. (3) There was a failure to provide longer range data. (4) Would results differ depending on the type of acellular dermal matrix used, and finally and ultimately will this really be the Holy Grail to prevent capsular contracture in humans?

S. H. Miller, MD

An Innovative Procedure for the Treatment of Primary and Recurrent Capsular Contracture (CC) Following Breast Augmentation

Costagliola M, Atiyeh BS, Rampillon F (Toulouse Univ, France; American Univ of Beirut Med Ctr, Lebanon; Dijon Univ, France)

Aesthet Surg J 33:1008-1017, 2013

Background.—Capsular contracture (CC) is the most frequently reported complication following alloplastic breast augmentation. At present, none of the available preventive measures are effective, and various treatment modalities have been advocated. Reduction of the inflammatory process is critical for successful treatment. Late intracapsular glucocorticosteroid (GC) injections have been somewhat effective for the treatment, but the fine balance between the effectiveness of therapeutic GC dosages and their potential serious side effects is of utmost importance.

Objectives.—The authors investigate whether instillation of a rapid-acting water-soluble GC in the implant pocket during the early proliferative phase of wound healing is more effective than delayed instillation during the remodeling phase.

Methods.—Between 2003 and 2009, 33 consecutive patients presenting with CC (Baker grades III and IV) were managed by capsulectomy with implant replacement and corticosteroid therapy immediately as well as 2 to 3 days later through an indwelling catheter left in place for that period. This delayed but early administration is a novel technique for GC injection.

Results.—Complete correction of the contracture with no recurrence was achieved in all patients with a follow-up range of 2 to 10 years.

Conclusions.—This GC administration technique avoids the potential complications of long-term, slow corticosteroid release. It has a targeted anti-inflammatory effect, probably at a critical stage of the healing process, and could effectively prevent CC following alloplastic breast augmentation.

▶ Prevention and treatment of capsular contracture (CC) after breast augmentation remains a challenge. Steroid injections into the breast implant pocket or steroid placement into saline implants can lead to serious complications and has been abandoned for many years. The authors, however, used Solu-Medrol® (Methylprednisolone Sodium Succinate), a short-acting steroid, instead of Kenalog® (Triamcinolone Acetonide), the longer-acting steroid used in the past. They do mention that one patient had early subcutaneous atrophy in the lower lateral breast quadrant, with bluish skin translucency, which resolved spontaneously within 6 months. Although these results appear promising, it may be premature to recommend widespread use of this technique. Because the authors also used an antibiotic irrigation, and most patients had replacement with textured implants, it is difficult to attribute the lack of CC recurrence to the steroid injection alone. Anyone considering this treatment for a patient with recurrent CC needs to provide a detailed informed consent regarding the potential risks involved (tissue thinning and implant extrusion). Because the authors state that they now use this technique prophylactically on all breast augmentations, it may be better to see a follow-up publication on the long-term results.

K. A. Gutowski, MD

Breast augmentation via the abdominoplasty incision approach: a prospective study of 100 cases

Dini GM, Milani J, Albuquerque LG, et al (Chief of the Rhinoplasty Sector of the Discipline of Plastic Surgery (UNIFESP-EPM), São Paulo, Brazil; Undergraduate Student of Medicine (UNIFESP-EPM), São Paulo, Brazil; Graduated at the City of São Paulo Univ (UNICID), Brazil; et al)
Rev Bras Cir Plást 28:105-113, 2013

Introduction.—Pregnancy and obesity cause distension of the abdominal wall and produce changes in the shape and size of the breasts. Thus, the need of aesthetic improvement of the abdominal area is not uncommon, coinciding with the desire for breast augmentation. Performing mammoplasty via the abdominoplasty incision approach was first described in 1976. Because of the lack of prospective studies using this approach, we performed a series of dermolipectomy procedures using the abdominal incision to insert a pair of silicone gel breast implants.

Methods.—In total, 100 consecutive patients were selected, with a mean age of 33 ± 2 years. Classic abdominoplasty was performed, and 2 tunnels were then made in the right and left hypochondria. After implant placement, the mammary fold was reconstructed using simple sutures with absorbable threads to attach the subcutaneous tissue to the aponeurosis.

Results.—None of the following complications were observed: deep-vein thrombosis, cardiorespiratory or anesthetic complications, skin necrosis, visible bleeding, hematoma, or clinically detectable infection. The volume of the implants ranged from 280 to 450 mL (median, 350 mL). The mean operation time was 116 minutes. Reoperation was not necessary in any of the cases. The monitoring period ranged from 9 to 84 months (mean, 36 months).

Conclusions.—Breast augmentation via the abdominoplasty incision approach was demonstrated to be a reliable and simple technique, providing a new, scar-free alternative to mammary surgical procedures.

► The desire to avoid a breast incision and scar is common in patients desiring breast augmentation. The availability of an abdominoplasty approach may be useful in patients who have minimal or no breast ptosis and who not require inframammary fold (IMF) adjustment. However, the downsides of this approach include the following:

1 Need for proper (longer) equipment
2 Need to reconstruct the IMF, which is disrupted during the abdominoplasty approach
3 Potential for bacterial contamination because of the site of the abdominoplasty incision
4 Difficulty with submuscular implant placement (only subglandular placement was done in this series)

Also, based on the results shown, there seemed to be a tendency for high-positioned implants, perhaps because of limited ability to adjust the IMF from this approach.

K. A. Gutowski, MD

Cancer and Reconstruction

Incidence of Surgical-Site Infection Is Not Affected by Method of Immediate Breast Reconstruction

Costa MA, Rommer E, Peric M, et al (Univ of Southern California, Los Angeles, CA)

Plast Reconstr Surg 132:20e-29e, 2013

Background.—To date, few large-scale studies have reported the incidence of surgical-site infection in women undergoing mastectomy with respect to the various methods of immediate breast reconstruction. This study assessed whether the reconstruction method was associated with the risk of surgical-site infection in these patients.

Methods.—Using the National Surgical Quality Improvement Program database, 9230 female patients undergoing mastectomy with immediate reconstruction from 2005 to 2009 were identified. Reconstruction was classified as autologous, prosthetic, or hybrid. The primary outcome was the incidence of surgical-site infection within 30 days of operation. Univariate and multivariate analyses were performed to derive the unadjusted and adjusted risk of surgical-site infection according to reconstruction method.

Results.—The overall rate of surgical-site infection was 3.53 percent (95 percent CI, 3.15 to 3.94 percent), with individual rates of 3.33 percent (95 percent CI, 2.93 to 3.76 percent) for prosthetic reconstruction, 4.88 percent (95 percent CI, 3.48 to 6.11 percent) for autologous reconstruction, and 2.19 percent (95 percent CI, 0.88 to 4.45 percent) for hybrid reconstruction. The adjusted odds ratio of surgical-site infection was 1.14 (95 percent CI, 0.83 to 1.58; $p = 0.42$) for autologous versus prosthetic methods and 0.59 (95 percent CI, 0.27 to 1.27; $p = 0.18$) for hybrid versus prosthetic methods.

Conclusions.—Although the risk of surgical-site infection in patients undergoing immediate reconstruction is highest with autologous and lowest with hybrid methods of reconstruction, the difference in infection risk was not statistically significant after adjustment for confounding factors. Thus, all methods of reconstruction are viable options with regard to risk for surgical-site infection.

▶ I believe this is an important study for several reasons, not the least of which is that plastic surgeons are beginning to use and evaluate large databases to address questions of importance to all plastic surgeons. The data demonstrate no "real statistically significant or important clinical difference" among breast reconstruction using implants, autologous tissue, or some combination for immediate reconstruction of the breast after mastectomy. Of course, caveats are necessary when reading this report: the difficulty of assuring accuracy in coding and recording of the data and the inability to check the accuracy of the data, the limitation of assessment to only 30 days postoperatively (some 20%–25% of infections do occur after the 30-day window), and the ultimate effect of infection on the outcome.

S. H. Miller, MD

The Influence of Dispositional Optimism on Decision Regret to Undergo Major Breast Reconstructive Surgery

Zhong T, Bagher S, Jindal K, et al (Univ Health Network, Toronto, Canada; Univ of Toronto, Canada; et al)
J Surg Oncol 108:526-530, 2013

Background & Objectives.—It is not known if optimism influences regret following major reconstructive breast surgery. We examined the relationship between dispositional optimism, major complications and decision regret in patients undergoing microsurgical breast reconstruction.

Methods.—A consecutive series of 290 patients were surveyed. Independent variables were: (1) dispositional optimism and (2) major complications. The primary outcome was Decision Regret. A multivariate regression analysis determined the relationship between the independent variables, confounders and decision regret.

Results.—Of the 181 respondents, 63% reported no regret after breast reconstruction, 26% had mild regret, and 11% moderate to severe regret. Major complications did not have a significant effect on decision regret, and the impact of dispositional optimism was not significant in Caucasian women. There was a significant effect in non-Caucasian women with less optimism who had significantly higher levels of mild regret 1.36 (CI 1.02–1.97) and moderate to severe regret 1.64 (CI 1.0–93.87).

Conclusions.—This is the first paper to identify a subgroup of non-Caucasian patients with low dispositional optimism who may be at risk for developing regret after microsurgical breast reconstruction. Possible strategies to ameliorate regret may involve addressing cultural and language barriers, setting realistic expectations, and providing more supports during the pre-operative decision-making phase.

► Plastic surgeons have always known that a certain percentage of the patients upon whom they operate will be unhappy or dissatisfied about the results achieved. Admonitions from our teachers/mentors and recognized leaders in the field have cautioned us to be careful in choosing patients and to be aware of red flag warnings that suggest we might be better off not agreeing to perform surgery for particular patients. Most often, these admonitions have been based on experience and instinct but without much evidence that our decisions are based on valid and reliable information. The current study, using an instrument called *Life Oriented Test-Revised*[1] to assess dispositional optimism/pessimism, seemed to detect a subgroup of patients, primarily nonwhites, likely to regret having undergone microsurgical breast reconstruction. It is of interest that the development of postoperative complications in this study was not associated with decision regret. The population studied was primarily white and centered on those who came to a single tertiary care center in Canada. The nonwhite group studied was quite small and could not be stratified further as to the specific racial groups. Finally, it is unclear if the same conclusions would hold for patients undergoing breast reconstruction using implants and patients who have not undergone reconstruction. Needless to say, other studies, in different centers and with different populations, will be needed to assess the reliability and validity of these findings and the research tool used for this study.

S. H. Miller, MD

Reference

1. Schou I, Ekeberg Ø, Ruland OM, Sandvik L, Kåresen R. Pessimism as a predictor of emotional morbidity one year following breast cancer surgery. *Psychooncology.* 2004;13:309-320.

Proton Therapy for Breast Cancer After Mastectomy: Early Outcomes of a Prospective Clinical Trial

MacDonald SM, Patel SA, Hickey S, et al (Massachusetts General Hosp, Boston)
Int J Radiat Oncol Biol Phys 86:484-490, 2013

Proton radiation is a form of particle radiation that allows for sparing of tissues distal to the target volume. Comparative planning studies for breast cancer patients suggest potential benefits for protons over standard radiation by improving target volume coverage and cardiopulmonary sparing. The entrance dose is higher for proton radiation, leading to some concern regarding skin tolerance. We report early outcomes in 12 women treated with postmastectomy proton radiation therapy on a prospective clinical trial.

Purpose.—Dosimetric planning studies have described potential benefits for the use of proton radiation therapy (RT) for locally advanced breast cancer. We report acute toxicities and feasibility of proton delivery for 12 women treated with postmastectomy proton radiation with or without reconstruction.

Methods and Materials.—Twelve patients were enrolled in an institutional review board-approved prospective clinical trial. The patients were assessed for skin toxicity, fatigue, and radiation pneumonitis during treatment and at 4 and 8 weeks after the completion of therapy. All patients consented to have photographs taken for documentation of skin toxicity.

Results.—Eleven of 12 patients had left-sided breast cancer. One patient was treated for right-sided breast cancer with bilateral implants. Five women had permanent implants at the time of RT, and 7 did not have

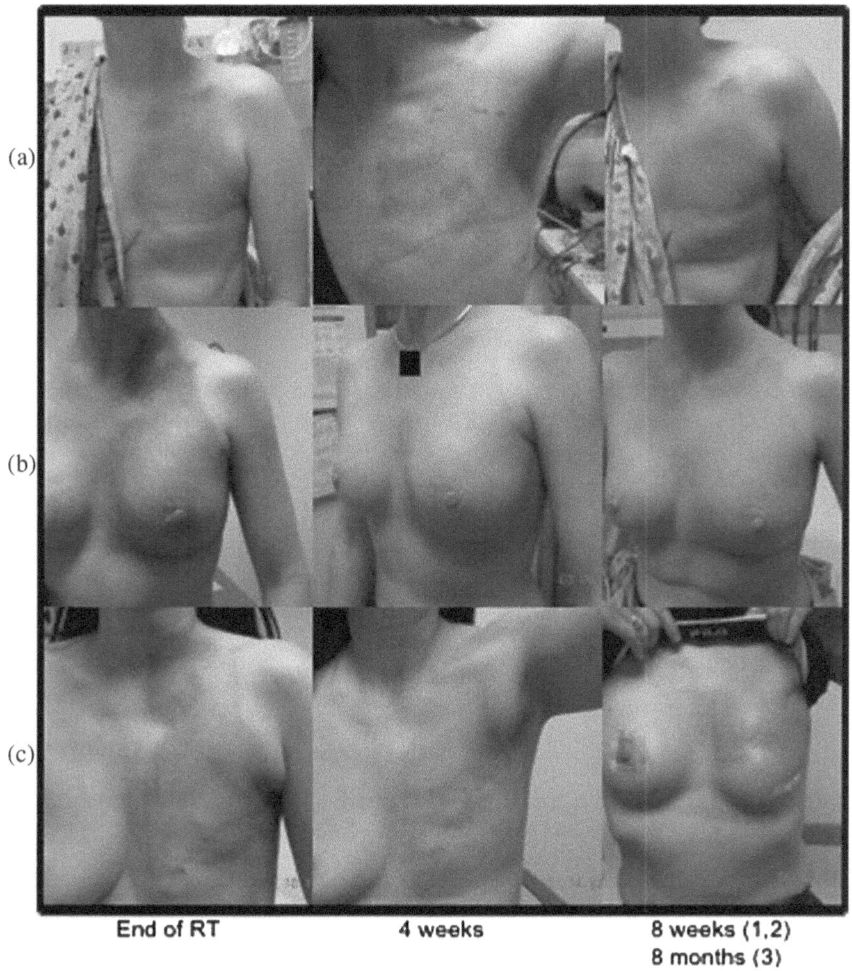

FIGURE 3.—Skin reactions at the end of proton radiation and after proton radiation for (a) a patient who underwent mastectomy without reconstruction, (b) a patient who underwent bilateral nipple-sparing mastectomy with permanent implants, and (c) a patient who underwent mastectomy without reconstruction followed by an expander/exchange reconstruction after radiation (last photo taken after surgery at 8-month follow-up visit). Figure depicts permanent implant. (Reprinted from MacDonald SM, Patel SA, Hickey S, et al. Proton therapy for breast cancer after mastectomy: early outcomes of a prospective clinical trial. *Int J Radiat Oncol Biol Phys*. 2013;86:484-490, with permission from Elsevier.)

immediate reconstruction. All patients completed proton RT to a dose of 50.4 Gy (relative biological effectiveness [RBE]) to the chest wall and 45 to 50.4 Gy (RBE) to the regional lymphatics. No photon or electron component was used. The maximum skin toxicity during radiation was grade 2, according to the Common Terminology Criteria for Adverse Events (CTCAE). The maximum CTCAE fatigue was grade 3. There have been no cases of RT pneumonitis to date.

Conclusions.—Proton RT for postmastectomy RT is feasible and well tolerated. This treatment may be warranted for selected patients with unfavorable cardiac anatomy, immediate reconstruction, or both that otherwise limits optimal RT delivery using standard methods (Fig 3).

▶ This is a small preliminary prospective study on the use of proton therapy for breast cancer after mastectomy. Apparently, proton therapy has not been reported for use to treat postmastectomy breast cancer. The primary purpose of this study, with a short-term follow-up, was to assess skin toxicity, fatigue, and radiation pneumonitis. Of interest to the plastic surgeon, however, is the fact that 5 patients had immediate reconstruction with implants and 1 patient had delayed implant reconstruction (Fig 3). The authors did not treat any patients with expander reconstruction or reconstruction with autogenous tissues. Overall, the results of this short-term study, from the standpoint of the radiation oncologist, were good. I am certain that interest in this type of radiation will grow. Whether this type of therapy will have a less detrimental effect on implant reconstruction remains to be seen.

S. H. Miller, MD

Breast sensibility after bilateral risk-reducing mastectomy and immediate breast reconstruction: A prospective study

Gahm J, Hansson P, Brandberg Y, et al (Karolinska Institutet, Stockholm, Sweden)

J Plast Reconstr Aesthet Surg 66:1521-1527, 2013

The demand for risk-reducing mastectomy (RRM) to avoid breast cancer has increased over the last several years, and knowledge of the outcome after this prophylactic surgical procedure is important. The primary aim of this study was to prospectively compare breast sensibility before and after RRM in a consecutive series of women. The study also investigated whether the nipples were less numb if the nipple areola complexes (NACs) were spared compared with regrafted nipple tips.

Forty-six women who selected bilateral RRM with immediate reconstruction using implants at the Karolinska University Hospital, Solna, Stockholm, Sweden, were included in the study. The median patient age at the time of surgery was 39 years (range 26–58). All patients were evaluated preoperatively and at least 2 years postoperatively (median 29 months). Tactile, thermal and nociceptive cutaneous sensibilities were studied with quantitative techniques. The patients at the postoperative evaluation completed a questionnaire about subjective feelings in both breasts.

The results showed that breast sensibility is significantly impaired after RRM. Additionally, the ability to experience sexual sensations in the breast is often lost. An NAC-sparing surgery did not result in better nipple sensibility.

▶ This is an interesting addition to the literature on the sensory ramifications of performing prophylactic, risk-reducing mastectomy (RRM in the authors' study). Removal, or destruction, of the median and lateral branches of the third through fifth intercostal nerves during the course of a prophylactic mastectomy has generally been accepted as an unavoidable downside to the procedure, and the authors clearly document that in this study. What is less clear is why the sensory loss was not universal in all of their patients; several actually having sensation comparable to their preoperative levels. Additionally, the authors report that the patients were less able to appreciate sexual feelings in the breast after this surgery, but these data are based on subjective patient evaluations coming many years after the procedure, and it was unclear if those patients who retained comparable preoperative levels of sensation also maintained the ability to appreciate sexual feelings in the breast.

S. H. Miller, MD

A Comparison of Acellular Dermal Matrix to Autologous Dermal Flaps in Single-Stage, Implant-Based Immediate Breast Reconstruction: A Cost-Effectiveness Analysis

Krishnan NM, Chatterjee A, Van Vliet MM, et al (Dartmouth Hitchcock Med Ctr, Hanover, NH; Tuck School of Business at Dartmouth, Lebanon, NH)

Plast Reconstr Surg 131:953-961, 2013

Background.—The use of acellular dermal matrix has allowed for single-stage immediate breast reconstruction after mastectomy at a significantly decreased cost compared with two-stage expander/implant reconstruction. The use of a pedicled autologous dermal flap in the same fashion as acellular dermal matrix in women with larger, ptotic breasts has also allowed for single-stage immediate breast reconstruction with similarly low complication rates and without the added procedural cost of using acellular dermal matrix. There have been no prior studies evaluating whether the added procedural cost for acellular dermal matrix is cost-effective relative to using an autologous dermal flap in single-stage immediate breast reconstruction following mastectomy.

Methods.—A comprehensive literature review was conducted to identify published complication rates for single-stage, implant-based immediate breast reconstruction using either acellular dermal matrix or an autologous dermal flap. The probabilities of the most common complications were combined with Medicare Current Procedural Terminology reimbursement codes and expert utility estimates to fit into a decision model to evaluate the cost-effectiveness of acellular dermal matrix.

Results.—The decision model revealed a baseline cost difference of \$261.72 and a 0.001 increase in the quality-adjusted life years when using acellular dermal matrix, yielding an incremental cost-utility ratio of $261,720 per quality-adjusted life year. Sensitivity analysis showed that acellular dermal matrix was not cost-effective when the complication rate for autologous dermal flaps was below 20 percent.

Conclusions.—The authors' study demonstrates that acellular dermal matrix is not a cost-effective technology in patients who can have an autologous dermal flap in single-stage immediate breast reconstruction.

▶ This is an elegant and sophisticated cost-effectiveness analysis comparing breast reconstruction using a sling of acellular dermal matrix (AlloDerm) with reconstruction creating a sling using an autologous pedicled dermal flap created by de-epithelializing the inferior mastectomy flap after performance of a mastectomy. The authors conclude that the use of acellular dermal matrix is not warranted if surgeons can perform reconstruction using the dermal flap technique with a complication rate of less than 20%. Of course, the point is moot in those patients whose body mass index is such that the breasts are not sufficiently large to allow harvesting such a flap. Having harvested dermis for many procedures from a variety of sites, one wonders if those patients who do not have adequate material to form an inferiorly based mastectomy flap could have fascia/dermis harvested from elsewhere and used to fashion a sling to accomplish one-stage breast reconstruction.

S. H. Miller, MD

Dermal autografts as a substitute for acellular dermal matrices (ADM) in tissue expander breast reconstruction: A prospective comparative study

Lynch MP, Chung MT, Rinker BD (Univ of Kentucky, Lexington; Univ of Kentucky College of Medicine, Lexington)

J Plast Reconstr Aesthet Surg 66:1534-1542, 2013

The use of acellular dermal matrix (ADM) in tissue expander breast reconstruction has several advantages but increased complications have been reported. Dermal autografts may offer a safer and more cost-effective alternative. The purpose of this prospective study was to compare the outcomes of tissue expander breast reconstruction using dermal autografts with ADM-assisted reconstruction. Patients undergoing tissue expander breast reconstruction with either ADM or dermal autografts were enrolled. Autografts were harvested from the lower abdomen. At each follow-up visit, patients were surveyed on a seven-point scale for scar and overall satisfaction. Biopsies taken at the time of device exchange were evaluated histologically with CD34 staining to assess tissue integration and vessel ingrowth. Expansion parameters, complications, procedural costs, and operative times were compared. Forty-eight patients were enrolled (76 breasts). Twenty-seven patients received ADM, and twenty-one patients received dermal autograft. Wound healing complications were significantly higher in the ADM group (14.8% versus 4.8%,

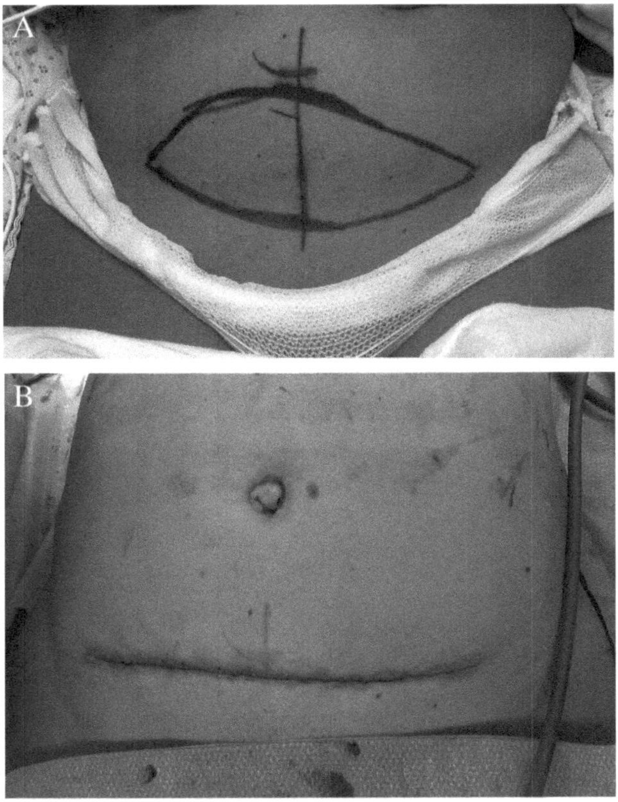

FIGURE 1.—(A) Preoperative and (B) postoperative photographs of a 45-year-old female patient who underwent tissue expander breast reconstruction with dermal autograft. The dermal autograft was harvested as a horizontally-oriented ellipse measuring 16 × 6-cm for unilateral reconstruction and 26 × 6-cm for bilateral reconstruction. (Reprinted from Journal of Plastic, Reconstructive & Aesthetic Surgery. Lynch MP, Chung MT, Rinker BD. Dermal autografts as a substitute for acellular dermal matrices (ADM) in tissue expander breast reconstruction: a prospective comparative study. *J Plast Reconstr Aesthet Surg*. 2013;66:1534-1542, Copyright 2013, with permission from British Association of Plastic, Reconstructive and Aesthetic Surgeons.)

p-value = 0.03), as were major complications (18.5% versus 0%, *p*-value < 0.01). Histologic vessel counts in the autograft group averaged 21 vessels/mm^2, compared to 7 vessels/mm^2 in the ADM group (*p*-value < 0.01). There was no difference between the two groups in scar satisfaction or overall satisfaction. Patients receiving dermal autograft had a lower incidence of major complications and delayed wound healing than patients who received ADM. Despite harvest time, the overall cost of the ADM-assisted expander placement was higher. Dermal autograft-assisted breast reconstruction offers many of the benefits of ADM, but with a lower cost and improved safety profile (Figs 1-3).

▶ It is obvious that the use of acellular dermal matrix for breast reconstruction, despite great enthusiasm when first introduced, is being carefully re-evaluated

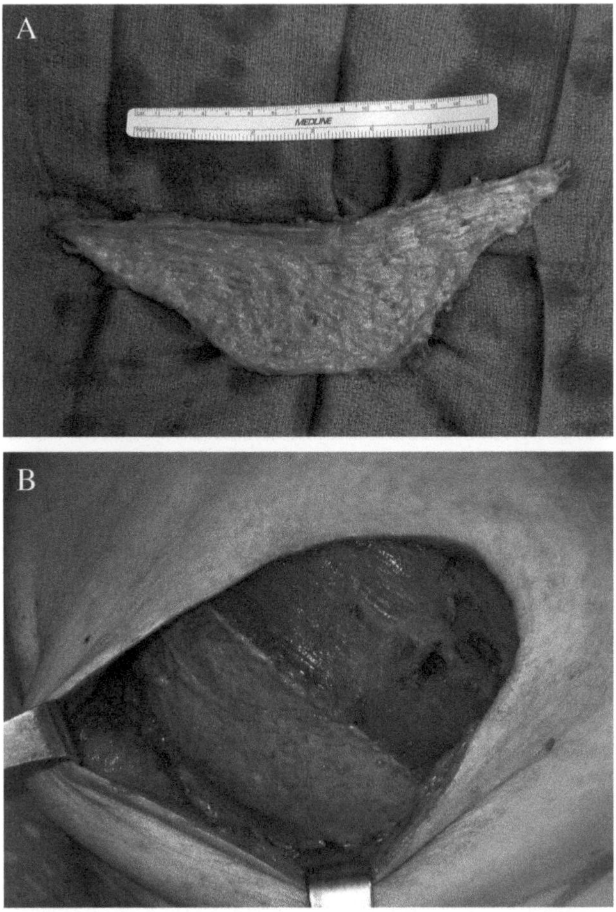

FIGURE 2.—(A) Intraoperative photograph of a 53-year-old female patient who underwent tissue expander breast reconstruction with dermal autograft. De-epithelialization and defatting was performed *in situ* on a back table. (B) The dermal autograft was then sutured, superficial side up, to the inframammary fold, lateral mammary fold, and inferior border of the pectoralis major muscle. (Reprinted from Journal of Plastic, Reconstructive & Aesthetic Surgery. Lynch MP, Chung MT, Rinker BD. Dermal autografts as a substitute for acellular dermal matrices (ADM) in tissue expander breast reconstruction: a prospective comparative study. *J Plast Reconstr Aesthet Surg*. 2013;66:1534-1542, Copyright 2013, with permission from British Association of Plastic, Reconstructive and Aesthetic Surgeons.)

in many different breast centers.[1] The high price/cost of the material and high incidence of complications seem to outweigh its convenience and alleged benefits. Most breast surgeons, be they of the reconstructive ilk or aesthetic variety, see the obvious benefits in total coverage of the breast implant with tissue/muscle other than the patient's own skin, especially in the lateral and inferior aspects of the pocket created for the implant. It is encouraging to me to see the creativity being used to find new solutions for the problem and greater attempts to study those solutions and report them in a less anecdotal manner. Clearly, this study is small and needs to be evaluated by others, especially in

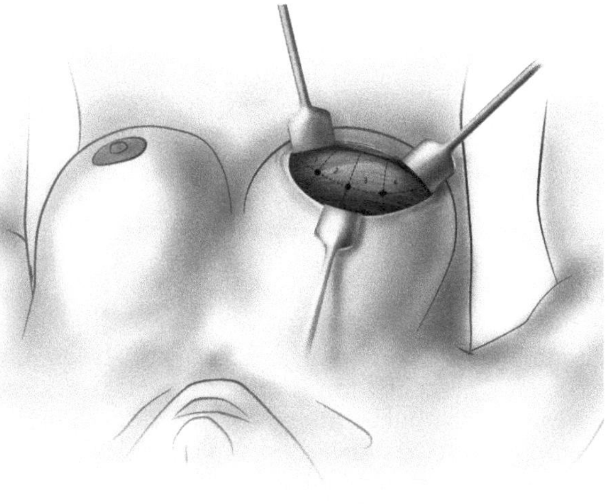

FIGURE 3.—At the time of expander implant exchange, three small samples of the internal capsule were harvested from standard locations, at the site of the previous ADM or autograft placement, with a 4-mm biopsy punch. (Reprinted from Journal of Plastic, Reconstructive & Aesthetic Surgery. Lynch MP, Chung MT, Rinker BD. Dermal autografts as a substitute for acellular dermal matrices (ADM) in tissue expander breast reconstruction: a prospective comparative study. *J Plast Reconstr Aesthet Surg*. 2013;66:1534-1542, Copyright 2013, with permission from British Association of Plastic, Reconstructive and Aesthetic Surgeons.)

randomized fashion, but also with greater numbers of patients so as to enable the data from the subgroup analysis to be more robust.

S. H. Miller, MD

Reference

1. Krishnan NM, Chatterjee A, Van Vliet MM, Powell SG, Rosen JM, Nigriny JF. A comparison of acellular dermal matrix to autologous dermal flaps in single-stage, implant-based immediate breast reconstruction: a cost-effectiveness analysis. *Plast Reconstr Surg*. 2013;131:953-961.

Analysis of the National Surgical Quality Improvement Program Database in 19,100 Patients Undergoing Implant-Based Breast Reconstruction: Complication Rates with Acellular Dermal Matrix

Ibrahim AMS, Shuster M, Koolen PGL, et al (Harvard Med School, Boston, MA)

Plast Reconstr Surg 132:1057-1066, 2013

Background.—The use of acellular dermal matrices has become increasingly popular in immediate and delayed tissue expander/implant-based breast reconstruction. However, it is unclear whether their use is associated with increased postoperative complication rates. Using the American College of Surgeons National Surgical Quality Improvement Program database, the authors assessed baseline differences in demographics and comorbidities with and without acellular dermal matrix and determined whether postoperative complication rates varied.

Methods.—Using the national surgical database (2005 to 2011), tissue expander/implant–based breast reconstruction cases were extracted using Current Procedural Terminology codes. Differences in preoperative demographics and comorbidities were assessed using chi-square and t test analysis using SPSS. The authors analyzed variations in complication rates and determined whether demographics and comorbidities affected outcomes using multivariate logistical analysis. A post hoc power study was calculated.

Results.—Of 19,100 cases, 3301 involved acellular dermal matrix use. Overall complication rates were not statistically significant (acellular dermal matrix, 5.3 percent; non–acellular dermal matrix, 4.9 percent; $p = 0.396$). Several risk factors were statistically significant associated factors of complications. Higher body mass index was associated with wound complications in both cohorts. In the non-acellular dermal matrix group, body mass index, smoking, and diabetes were associated with major complications, and radiotherapy and steroid use with minor complications.

Conclusions.—Acellular dermal matrix use did not appear to increase complication rates in tissue expander/implant-based breast reconstruction in this survey of a national surgical database. There was no significant difference in complication rates between the acellular dermal matrix and non–acellular dermal matrix groups.

Clinical Question/Level of Evidence.—Therapeutic, III.

▶ This is a much-welcomed study documenting the differences in some complication rates after breast reconstruction using acellular dermal matrix (ADM) and breast reconstructions without ADM based on data accumulated from the American College of Surgeons National Surgical Quality Improvement Program (NSQIP) databases from 2005 through 2011. The authors report no appreciable differences in rates of complications regardless of whether ADM was used, but according to data reported in Table 3 of the original article, the ADM group did have a statistically higher incidence of superficial wound infection. I was unable to find documentation of the incidence of seroma in this report. In both groups studied, higher body mass index was associated with greater numbers of wound complications. It is of interest that higher body mass index has been reported as a risk factor in other plastic surgical reports of complications after breast surgery but not in patients who underwent major thoracic, abdominal, or pelvic surgery for cancer.[1] Of course, the NSQIP data are currently the best we have, but in my mind it needs to be massaged a bit to make it more relevant for plastic surgery. For instance, most plastic surgeons and their patients are interested in longer-term follow-ups and outcomes beyond acute postoperative problems.

S. H. Miller, MD

Reference

1. Al-Refaie WB, Parsons HM, Henderson WG, et al. Body mass index and major cancer surgery outcomes: lack of association or need for alternative measurement of obesity. *Ann Surg Oncol.* 2010;17:2264-2273.

Beyond Biologics: Absorbable Mesh as a Low-Cost, Low-Complication Sling for Implant-Based Breast Reconstruction

Tessler O, Reish RG, Maman DY, et al (Massachusetts General Hosp, Boston)
Plast Reconstr Surg 133:90e-99e, 2014

Background.—There is an intense push to decrease overall healthcare costs in the United States. Although the use of acellular dermal matrix in implant-based reconstruction has grown significantly over the past decade, potential drawbacks remain a source of debate. Matrices are costly and not universally available across institutions, whereas Vicryl mesh is widely available, relatively inexpensive, and resistant to bacteria biofilm formation. With the intent of maximizing the reconstructive and economic advantages of direct-to-implant breast reconstruction, the authors report the first experience in the literature using an absorbable mesh as an inferolateral sling.

Methods.—A retrospective review was performed of the first 50 consecutive patients (76 reconstructions) who underwent implant-based breast reconstruction with Vicryl mesh from August of 2011 until June of 2012.

Results.—Fifty patients underwent 76 direct-to-implant reconstructions with Vicryl mesh between August of 2011 and June of 2012 (mean follow-up, 1.2 years). Five breasts (6.6 percent) had complications, with only one complication resulting in implant loss (1.3 percent). Implant positioning and contour were excellent, with only two patients [three breasts (3.9 percent)] undergoing revision procedures, for size enlargement. Using costs available at the authors' institution, use of Vicryl mesh instead of acellular dermal matrix resulted in a direct material cost savings of $172,112 in 10 months.

Conclusions.—Results to date have been encouraging, with a low complication rate (6.6 percent) and excellent aesthetic results. The technique has resulted in $172,112 in direct material cost savings over 10 months. Continued follow-up is planned to evaluate long-term results.

Clinical Question/Level of Evidence.—Therapeutic, IV.

▶ In this preliminary retrospective review with a short follow-up (average follow-up of 1.2 years), the authors suggest that the use of Vicryl mesh is a good, low-cost alternative to the use of acellular dermal matrix for immediate breast reconstruction. The concept of using absorbable mesh, rather than acellular dermal matrix, for immediate breast reconstruction is not a novel concept. Several authors have promoted the use of these nonbiologic products in the past using a product (TIGR) that is more costly but longer lasting than Vicryl.[1] Clearly additional study is needed, as are meaningful comparisons of costs, risks (infection, seroma, etc), and short- and long-term outcomes, including patient satisfaction, achieved using biologic materials (acellular dermal matrices of various types) compared with nonbiologic mesh (Vicryl, TIGR) to provide patients and providers with the knowledge necessary to enable informed decisions. Does the use of a longer-lasting nonbiologic absorbable material provide better results and justify their increased cost?

S. H. Miller, MD

Reference

1. Becker H, Lind JG. The use of synthetic mesh in reconstructive, revision, and cosmetic breast surgery. *Aesthetic Plast Surg*. 2013;37:914-921.

Implant-Based Breast Reconstruction Using a Titanium-Coated Polypropylene Mesh (TiLOOP Bra): A Multicenter Study of 231 Cases

Dieterich M, Paepke S, Zwiefel K, et al (Univ of Rostock, Germany; Technische Universität München, Germany; Univ of Düsseldorf, Germany; et al)
Plast Reconstr Surg 132:8e-19e, 2013

Background.—An alternative to implant-based breast reconstruction using acellular dermal matrix is the use of a titanium-coated polypropylene mesh. The mesh was approved for implant-based breast reconstruction in Europe in 2008, but only limited clinical data are available.

Methods.—Two hundred seven patients (231 breasts) with skin-sparing/nipple-sparing or modified radical mastectomy and immediate or delayed implant-based breast reconstruction using titanium-coated polypropylene mesh were evaluated retrospectively. The primary endpoints were identification of patient-related and surgical factors that were predictive for an adverse outcome and the development of recommendations for patients eligible for implant-based breast reconstruction using the mesh. Complications were divided into major (need for additional surgery), minor (conservative treatment), and implant loss. Univariate and multivariate logistic regression analyses were performed to determine the influence of the patient- and procedure-related characteristics on postoperative complications and implant loss.

Results.—No risk factors were observed for patient-associated complications. Major complications occurred in 13.4 percent, minor complications in 15.6 percent, and implant loss in 8.7 percent of patients. Univariate analysis revealed procedure-related risk factors for postoperative complications with a bilateral procedure ($p = 0.013$) or skin expansion before implant surgery ($p = 0.043$). Multivariate analysis confirmed these risk factors and revealed an increased risk for implant loss in patients with skin necrosis ($p < 0.001$) and capsule fibrosis ($p < 0.001$).

Conclusions.—This titanium-coated polypropylene mesh shows acceptable complication rates and can be a helpful device in implant-based breast

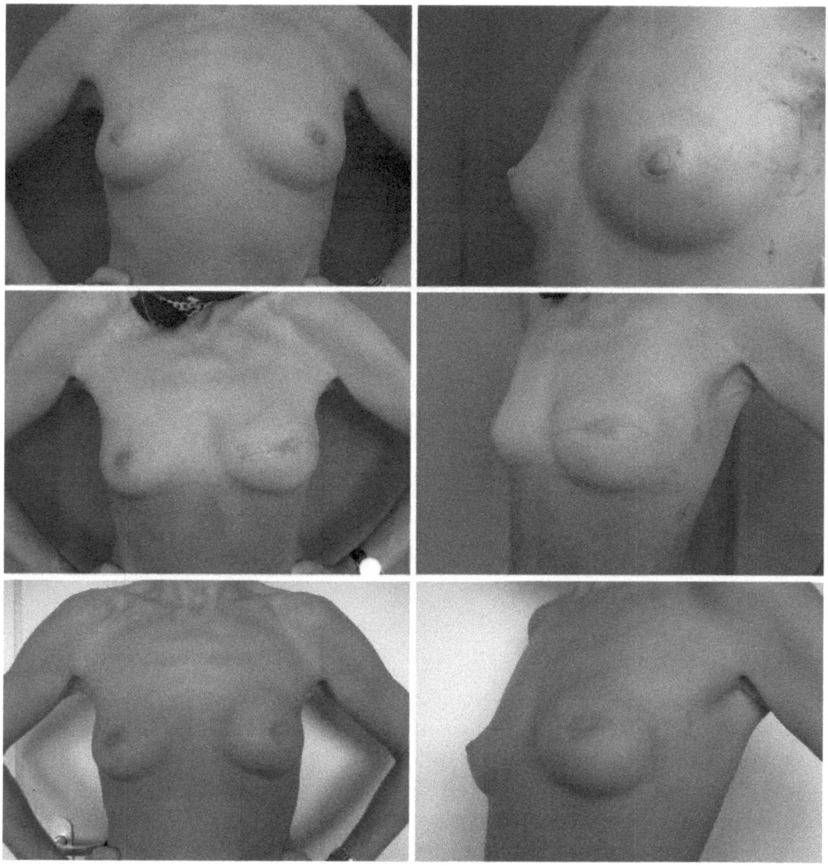

FIGURE 3.—(*Above, left*) Invasive breast cancer (left breast) with accompanying ductal carcinoma in situ after breast-conserving attempt (before skin-sparing mastectomy). (*Above, right*) Before skin-sparing mastectomy, oblique view. Immediately after skin-sparing mastectomy and implant-based breast reconstruction with titanium-coated polypropylene mesh, frontal (*center, left*) and oblique (*center, right*) views. Left breast 6 months postoperatively, frontal (*below, left*) and oblique (*below, right*) views. (Reprinted from Dieterich M, Paepke S, Zwiefel K, et al. Implant-based breast reconstruction using a titanium-coated polypropylene mesh (TiLOOP Bra): a multicenter study of 231 cases. *Plast Reconstr Surg*. 2013;132:8e-19e, with permission from American Society of Plastic Surgeons.)

reconstruction. The mesh should only be used in primary cases and, when adhering to the proposed indications, is a safe and convenient option in implant-based breast reconstruction.

Clinical Question/Level of Evidence.—Risk, III (Figs 3 and 4).

► A somewhat different approach to immediate breast reconstruction is presented in this retrospective multicenter study from several centers for breast surgery in Germany. This material is not approved for use in the United States. In reading between the lines, one gets the impression that the primary motivation for use of the titanium-coated polypropylene mesh was the much greater cost,

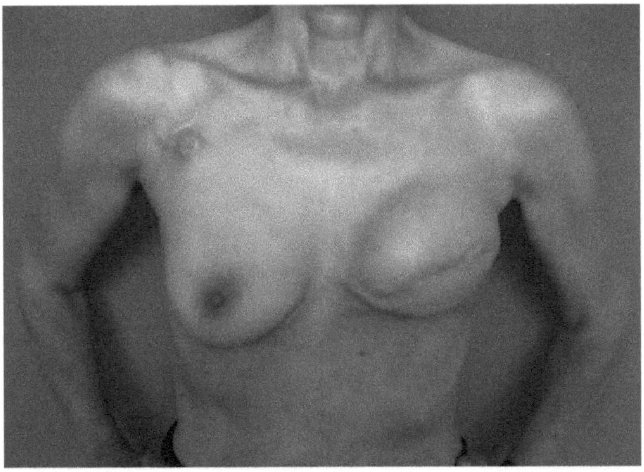

FIGURE 4.—Patient after modified radical mastectomy who desired secondary breast reconstruction. With a body mass index of 19 kg/m^2, she was not a candidate for autologous reconstruction. The surgical procedure was complex, with an elevation of the inframammary fold and mobilization of a thoracoepigastric flap. The implant had to be removed 3 months later. (Reprinted from Dieterich M, Paepke S, Zwiefel K, et al. Implant-based breast reconstruction using a titanium-coated polypropylene mesh (TiLOOP Bra): a multicenter study of 231 cases. *Plast Reconstr Surg.* 2013;132:8e-19e, with permission from American Society of Plastic Surgeons.)

in Europe, for acellular dermis. Likely, this increased cost makes it less likely that a true prospective comparison between the titanium mesh and acellular dermis would take place unless a multicenter study included centers in the countries in which acellular dermis is being used. It is interesting that the use of this material seems contraindicated in patients undergoing secondary reconstructions, possibly contraindicated in thin patients and/or patients with thin mastectomy flaps, in patients who underwent modified radical mastectomy, and patients scheduled to undergo radiation therapy. The follow-up time was relatively short. Clearly, although this material has possible uses, as in the case of acellular dermis, long-term risk-benefit and cost analyses should be performed.

S. H. Miller, MD

Evaluation of Pedicled Omental Flap Delivered through a Minilaparotomy for Immediate Breast Reconstruction in Obese Patients

Khater A (Mansoura Univ, Egypt)
Aesthetic Plast Surg 37:1140-1145, 2013

Background.—Studies have shown the laparoscopically harvested omental flap to be a successful method for immediate breast reconstruction. However, data about its usefulness and safety in obese women are limited. This study examined the effectiveness and safety of a pedicled omental flap delivered via a minilaparotomy in women with a body mass index (BMI) higher than 30 kg/m^2.

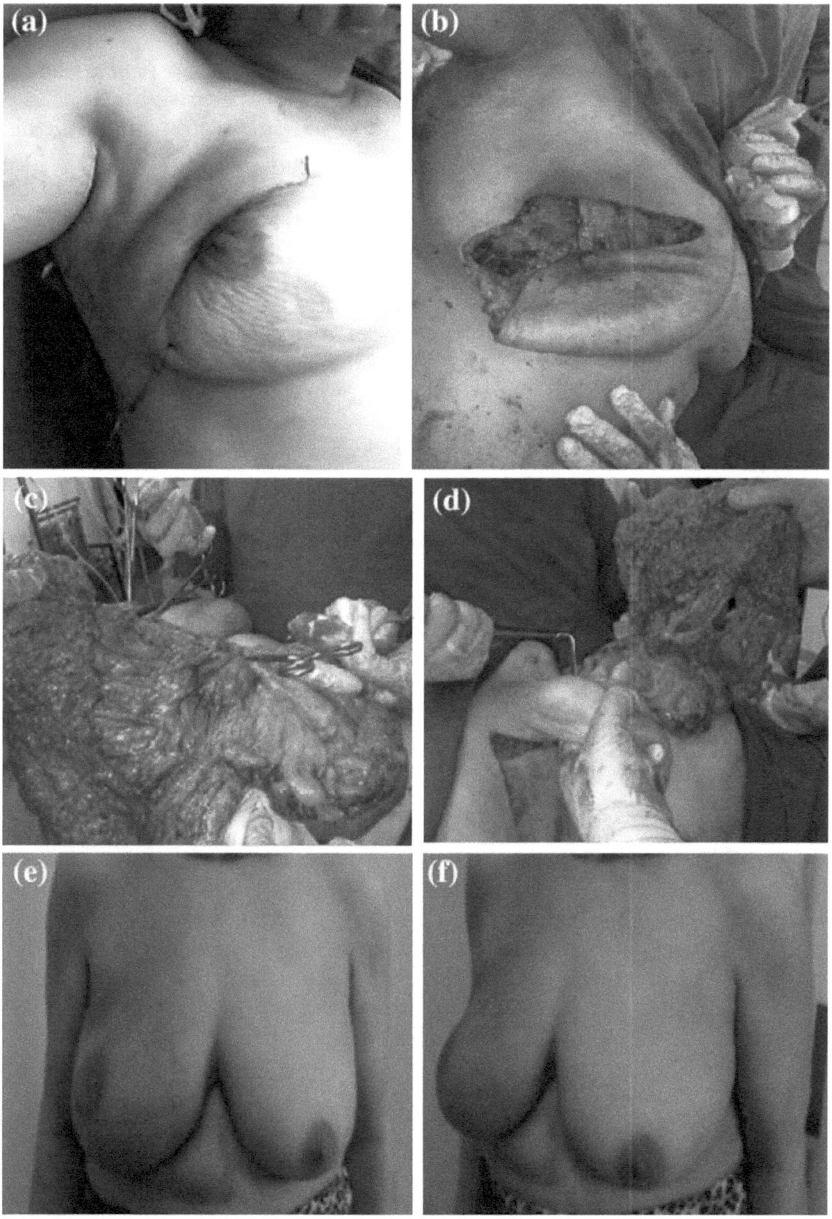

FIGURE 1.—A case of previously excised mass treated by nipplesparing mastectomy and pedicled omental flap reconstruction. **a** Preoperative view showing the scar of the excisional surgery. **b** Operative bed after mastectomy. c Extraction of the omentum via a minilaparotomy with clamping of the left gastroepiploic vessels. **d** Delivery of the omentum to the bed through the tunnel. **e** Front view eight months postoperatively showing the size gain phenomenon and excellent ptosis. **f** Side view of the same patient. (With kind permission from Springer Science+Business Media. Khater A. Evaluation of pedicled omental flap delivered through a minilaparotomy for immediate breast reconstruction in obese patients. *Aesthetic Plast Surg.* 2013;37:1140-1145, with permission from Springer Science+Business Media New York and International Society of Aesthetic Plastic Surgery.)

Methods.—Women candidates for skin-sparing mastectomy underwent reconstruction with delivery of a pedicled omental flap via a minilaparotomy.

Results.—Surgery was performed for 24 women with a mean age of 57.54 years and a mean BMI of 32.54 kg/m^2. The operative time was prolonged by about 1 h without excess blood loss or prolongation of their hospital stay. Except for a single case of partial flap necrosis, no single total flap loss was recorded. In three patients (12.5 %), the flap volume was inadequate, and silicone implant was used as an adjunct. Only one patient (4 %) experienced a small incisional hernia. The majority of the patients (67 %) described their cosmetic outcome as excellent.

Conclusion.—Delivery of a pedicled omental flap via a minilaparotomy is a safe and reliable method for immediate breast reconstruction after skin-sparing mastectomy in women with a BMI higher than 30 kg/m^2.

Level of Evidence V.—This journal requires that authors assign a level of evidence to each article. For a full description of these Evidence-Based Medicine ratings, please refer to the Table of Contents or the online Instructions to Authors www.springer.com/00266 (Fig 1).

▶ Surprising findings in obese patients! Many studies have clearly documented a significant increase in complications at the donor and recipient sites after breast reconstruction in obese patients.[1] In this small, prospective, and somewhat selective study, the author has compiled an excellent series of breast reconstructions using a pedicled omental flap, harvested via a minilaparotomy, in obese patients undergoing skin-sparing mastectomy. The primary complications related to breast asymmetry are no doubt caused by the large size of the retained breast as well as the variation in the volume of the harvested omentum over the course of time. Three patients required the use of a silicone implant to supplement the volume achieved with the use of the omentum alone. In these obese patients, I am sure that breast-balancing surgery, that is, breast reduction of the nonmastectomy breast, might also improve the cosmetic appearance. The results in the small number of patients (6 of 24) who underwent postoperative radiation therapy are not adequate to really assess the effects of that treatment on the results achieved. Overall, in the appropriate obese patient undergoing skin-sparing mastectomy, this method of reconstruction does merit consideration (Fig 1). One wonders whether this might also be true for the patient undergoing a unilateral prophylactic mastectomy?

S. H. Miller, MD

Reference

1. Ozturk CN, Kundu N, Bernard S, Cooper K, Ozturk C, Djohan R. Breast reconstruction with abdominal-based free flaps in high body mass index population. *Ann Plast Surg*. 2014;72:13-22.

Breast Reconstruction With Abdominal-Based Free Flaps in High Body Mass Index Population: Postoperative Complications and Impact of Weight Loss

Ozturk CN, Kundu N, Bernard S, et al (Cleveland Clinic, OH)
Ann Plast Surg 72:13-22, 2014

Obesity, which is becoming endemic in the United States, causes a significant challenge for reconstructive surgeons. This study evaluates postoperative complications and impact of weight loss in the high body mass index (BMI) population undergoing breast reconstruction with abdominal free flaps. A retrospective review of 182 consecutive patients was performed. Patients were divided into groups according to their BMI at the time of surgery (preoperative BMI) and presence of weight loss, and data were compared among groups. Multivariate analysis of effect of preoperative BMI on complications revealed that overall flap ($P = 0.008$) and donor ($P = 0.016$) complication rates were significantly higher in the obese

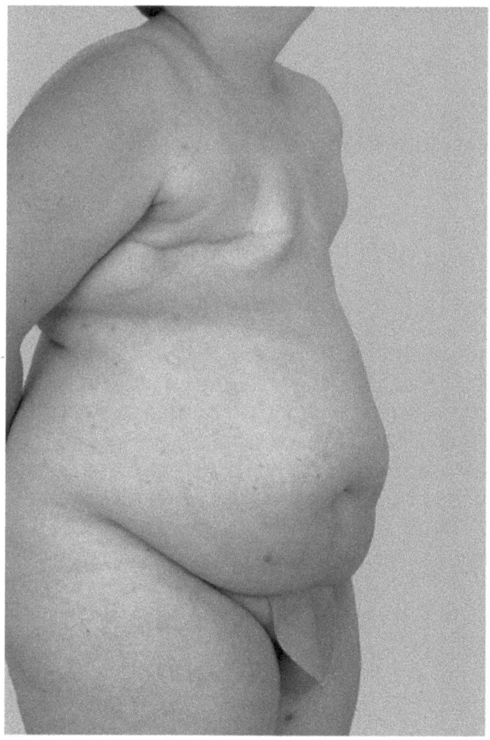

FIGURE 12.—Oblique view of patient. (Reprinted from Ozturk CN, Kundu N, Bernard S, et al. Breast reconstruction with abdominal-based free flaps in high body mass index population: Postoperative complications and impact of weight loss. *Ann Plast Surg*. 2014;72:13-22, with permission from Lippincott Williams & Wilkins.)

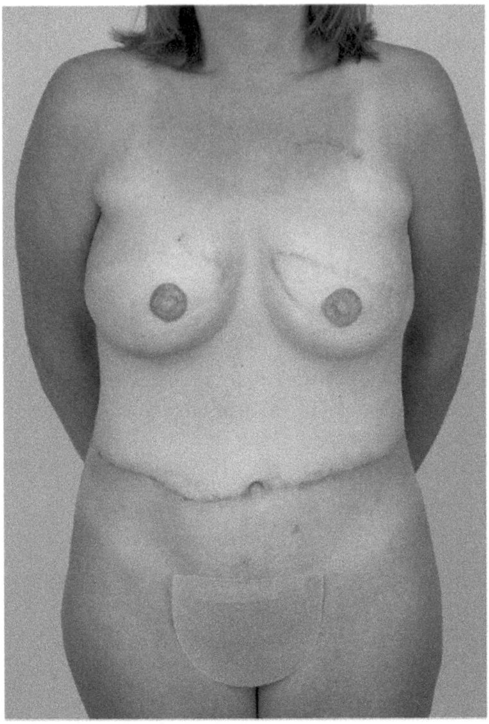

FIGURE 13.—BMI was reduced to 26.6 kg/m^2 at the time of DIEP surgery. Picture of patient after completion of bilateral nipple reconstructions and tattooing of areola. (Reprinted from Ozturk CN, Kundu N, Bernard S, et al. Breast reconstruction with abdominal-based free flaps in high body mass index population: Postoperative complications and impact of weight loss. *Ann Plast Surg*. 2014;72:13-22, with permission from Lippincott Williams & Wilkins.)

group. Analysis of preoperative weight loss did not yield a statistically significant reduction in flap ($P = 0.5161$) or donor ($P = 0.8034$) complication rates. Univariate analysis showed that higher preoperative BMI is associated with higher risk of systemic complications ($P = 0.027$). It is important to inform patients preoperatively that weight loss, although beneficial for ease of procedure and quality of life, does not diminish their increased risk of complications. Body mass index during surgery is the most important predictor of complications (Figs 12-14).

▶ This is an interesting study discussing the increased risks of free-flap reconstruction, primarily using deep inferior epigastric perforator flaps, after mastectomy in the obese patient. At the outset, I was struck by the fact that 264 free flaps were performed, 182 in therapeutic mastectomy patients and 77 in prophylactic mastectomy patients, but no further information is provided about the prophylactic mastectomy patient population as to status of their preoperative/postoperative weight or outcome. None of the results are particularly surprising aside from the fact that loss of weight before reconstruction seemed to

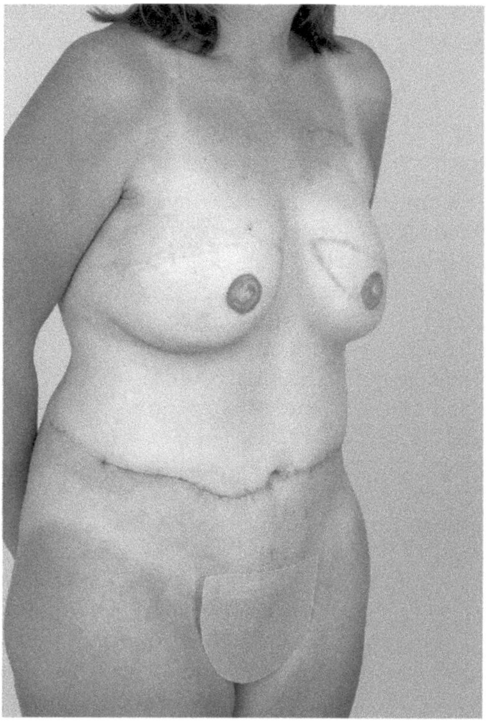

FIGURE 14.—Oblique view of patient. (Reprinted from Ozturk CN, Kundu N, Bernard S, et al. Breast reconstruction with abdominal-based free flaps in high body mass index population: Postoperative complications and impact of weight loss. *Ann Plast Surg*. 2014;72:13-22, with permission from Lippincott Williams & Wilkins.)

have no to little effect on the risk for complications. However, as stated, the amount of weight loss achieved in most of the patients in this study failed to place them in the normal body mass index (BMI) category. Also unclear is whether the duration of the weight loss, 12 months, was sufficient to allow the patients to have achieved a stable BMI. Finally, the numbers of patients in several of the subgroups were quite small, and the study was primarily a short-term one; thus, the data gleaned may not be of sufficient power to provide strong conclusions, especially with regard to smoking and postoperative radiation. Despite these problems, the results are actually quite good and confirm the author's contention that, although obesity is a risk factor for breast reconstruction, it is not an absolute contraindication (Figs 12-14).

S. H. Miller, MD

Processes of Care in Autogenous Breast Reconstruction with Pedicled TRAM Flaps: Expediting Postoperative Discharge in an Ambulatory Setting

Davidge KM, Brown M, Morgan P, et al (Univ of Toronto, Ontario, Canada; Womens College Hosp, Toronto, Ontario, Canada)

Plast Reconstr Surg 132:339e-344e, 2013

Background.—A multidisciplinary patient care plan was developed to facilitate early discharge following autogenous breast reconstruction and included (1) preadmission patient education, (2) perioperative multimodal pain management, (3) intraoperative nerve blocks, and (4) postdischarge telephone advice. This study evaluated the success of this care plan in the first 18 months after its implementation.

Methods.—A retrospective cohort study of all consecutive women undergoing pedicled transverse rectus abdominis myocutaneous (TRAM) flap breast reconstruction (November of 2009 to May of 2011) was performed. The primary outcome was time to discharge; secondary outcomes included complications, readmission, and self-report pain at discharge. Predictors of discharge time were analyzed using stepwise multivariable regression modeling.

Results.—Ninety-one women (mean age, 50.0 ± 8.5 years) underwent pedicled TRAM flap reconstruction (76 percent unilateral and 81 percent delayed), with 77 percent receiving the intended multimodal analgesia protocol. Mean time to discharge was 38.7 ± 27.6 hours. Overall, 40 percent of patients were discharged within 24 hours, but successful early discharge increased significantly over the study period. Key predictors of shorter time to discharge were use of multimodal analgesia, lower American Society of Anesthesiologists class, and surgery more than 6 months after implementation of the care plan.

Conclusions.—The authors' initial experience has supported the safety and feasibility of expedited discharge following pedicled TRAM flap breast reconstruction, with adherence to the authors' care plan improving steadily over the study period. Multimodal pain management proved a key modifiable factor in facilitating early discharge. A prospective study is currently underway to evaluate patient-reported quality of recovery following ambulatory surgery in this population.

▶ This is an important study for several reasons. The authors are to be congratulated for looking at patients from the standpoint of the ideal outcomes, such as time of discharge after surgery, optimal perioperative pain management after breast reconstruction using a pedicled TRAM flap, and patient postoperative experiences. Attention to detail regarding perioperative care specifically with regard to multimodality plans for pain management is obviously a key factor in the positive outcome. However, equally important, in my view, has been the decision to establish a goal and to continue to persist with the result that opioid use markedly decreased and the number of discharges within 24 hours of surgery also markedly increased from some 14% at the outset of the study to 83% at its conclusion. This is an excellent retrospective pilot study during which many parameters and therapies were explored to determine which were most efficacious. I think a much larger prospective study using the protocols developed by these authors, possibly involving other centers and reporting not only time of discharge and opioid use but patient experience, would be most welcome. One must wonder how many other areas of plastic surgical practice could also benefit from this type of study and data accumulation.

S. H. Miller, MD

Chronic Pain Following Abdominal Free Flap Breast Reconstruction: A Prospective Pilot Analysis

Nelson JA, Fischer JP, Pasick C, et al (Univ of Pennsylvania, Philadelphia; et al)

Ann Plast Surg 71:278-282, 2013

Background.—Chronic pain after breast reconstruction is an ill-defined process which can generate significant patient morbidity and disability. The purpose of this study was to examine chronic, persistent pain in a prospective study of free flap breast reconstruction patients, in an effort to identify possible points of intervention and counseling.

Methods.—We performed a prospective study evaluating function, quality of life, and satisfaction in patients undergoing abdominally based autologous reconstruction between 2006 and 2010. Using the short form 36, we examined the presence of chronic body pain (>4 months) as well as overall mental and physical health. Patients with debilitating pain were compared to those without in a post hoc analysis.

Results.—Overall, 399 women underwent reconstruction during the study period, with 149 enrolling and having long-term follow-up in this portion of the prospective study. Twenty-six (17%) of 149 patients experienced chronic body pain that was moderately debilitating after autologous reconstruction, making it one of the most common complications experienced in this cohort. No differences were noted in demographics, medical history, procedure type, history of axillary surgery, radiation treatment, surgical outcomes, or follow-up time between the cohorts. However, patients with chronic pain were found to have higher preoperative pain scores ($P < 0.0001$) and lower physical, mental, and overall health scores across time points. All scores significantly worsened with time in comparison to the cohort without pain, who, in contrast showed score improvement across all areas. Although pain issues trended toward being noted in postoperative visits more frequently in the chronic pain cohort (37% vs 19%, $P = 0.051$), only 1 (4.2%) patient was referred for pain service consultation. Additionally, satisfaction with reconstruction was significantly lower in patients who demonstrated chronic pain ($P = 0.03$).

Conclusions.—Factors contributing to chronic pain continue to be elusive and understudied. Our data demonstrate the importance of screening for chronic pain, as we determined that preoperative pain is linked to increased, moderately debilitating postoperative chronic pain. Persistent chronic pain, in turn, is associated with significant morbidity, disability, and dissatisfaction. Such patients with pain issues may benefit from additional preoperative counseling and early involvement of the pain service.

▶ Chronic pain after mastectomy without breast reconstruction occurs very frequently, with prevalence between 25% and 50%. In this prospective series of autologous breast reconstructions, it is difficult if not impossible to discern whether and if and how much the autologous reconstruction contributed to the development of chronic pain. One major fallacy is that the authors did not distinguish between chronic pain involving the breast or chest and chronic pain in general. They did, however, identify something potentially worthwhile to explore in greater detail. The 26 patients who had a diagnosis of chronic pain after mastectomy and autologous reconstruction had significant chronic pain preoperatively, pain which interfered with their work and contributed to lower physical and mental health scores and lower short form 36 (SF-36) scores. All of these scores worsened with time after mastectomy. Equally concerning is that most of these patients were dissatisfied with their reconstructions. The authors rightly do suggest that treatment needs to be a multimodality one postoperatively, but their suggestion that preoperative exercises to build up the abdominal musculature may be useful seems a bit naive. These patients require more extensive efforts to better understand their pre- and postoperative mental state as it relates to pain tolerance.[1]

S. H. Miller, MD

Reference

1. Wallace MS, Wallace AM, Lee J, Dobke MK. Pain after breast surgery: a survey of 282 women. *Pain.* 1996;66:195-205.

7 Grafts, Flaps, and Microsurgery

Scars

Analysis of Surgical Treatments for Earlobe Keloids: Analysis of 174 Lesions in 145 Patients

Ogawa R, Huang C, Akaishi S, et al (Nippon Med School, Tokyo, Japan; Nippon Med School Hosp, Tokyo, Japan)

Plast Reconstr Surg 132:818e-825e, 2013

Background.—Treatments for earlobe keloids include surgical excision, postoperative radiotherapy, steroid injection, taping stabilization, and pressure therapy. However, to date, there is no universally accepted treatment strategy for earlobe keloid therapy.

Methods.—A total of 174 lesions in 145 patients who attended the keloid/scar specialist clinic at the Department of Plastic, Reconstructive, and Aesthetic Surgery, Nippon Medical School, between 2006 and 2011 were included and were classified as having primary keloids or recurring keloids. Mild scars, such as hypertrophic scars, were excluded from this study. Appropriate surgical approaches, postoperative adjuvant therapies, such as radiotherapy, and postsurgical self-management were applied. The postsurgical radiotherapy modalities were 15 Gy administered in three fractions over 3 days and 10 Gy administered in two fractions over 2 days. Recurrence during the following 18-month follow-up period was recorded.

Results.—Of the 174 lesions, 85.6 percent were primary keloids and 14.4 percent were recurrent keloids. Their recurrence rates were 4.7 percent and 0 percent, respectively. The overall recurrence rate was 4.0 percent. Complications during the 18-month follow-up period were not observed. The groups treated with 15-Gy and 10-Gy postsurgical radiotherapy did not differ significantly in terms of recurrence rate ($p > 0.05$).

Conclusions.—Earlobe keloids can be treated by customized plans that involve appropriate surgical modalities, postoperative radiotherapy, and self-management. Postsurgical radiotherapy with 10 Gy of radiotherapy administered in two fractions over 2 days can be used successfully to treat earlobe keloids.

Clinical Question/Level of Evidence.—Therapeutic, IV.

▶ The authors report a very low recurrence rate after treating primary earlobe keloids (149 lesions, 4% to 7% recurrence) and recurrent earlobe keloids (25 lesions, 0% recurrence after treatment with 10 Gy postsurgical radiation). Postoperative radiation was fractionated over 2 days and compared with a dose of 15 Gy delivered in fractionated doses over 3 days. The latter did not appreciably improve the results, thus, accounting for their recommendation. Care was taken to shield uninvolved tissues from radiation. They also requested their patients try to prevent repeated injury to the earlobe by avoiding ear piercing and wearing surgical tape (silicone variety is preferable) for the first 6 months at night to prevent friction from pillows. Whether the latter works by direct protection or by exerting pressure on the earlobe was not addressed. Having seen examples and using some of these same techniques during my tenure in East Africa, I question if 18-month follow-up is adequate. It is possible that the radiation is delaying rather than preventing recurrence.

S. H. Miller, MD

Grafts

Prospective Randomized Controlled Trial: Fibrin Sealant Reduces Split Skin Graft Donor-Site Pain

Healy C, Greig AVH, Murphy AD, et al (St. Thomas' Hosp, London, UK; Imperial College London, UK)
Plast Reconstr Surg 132:139e-146e, 2013

Background.—Pain at split skin graft donor sites is common. Fibrin sealant has been demonstrated to reduce time to hemostasis at wound sites, and patients receiving this treatment were incidentally noted to report less pain. This study aimed to evaluate pain and incapacity in split skin graft donor sites treated with and without fibrin sealant.

Methods.—Fifty patients requiring thigh donor-site split skin grafts were prospectively randomized to receive either a self-adhesive fabric dressing alone or fibrin sealant plus the self-adhesive fabric dressing as primary donor-site dressings. External secondary dressings were the same. Patients were blinded with regard to treatment group. Using visual analogue scales (scored 0 to 5), patients rated their donor-site pain and incapacity for 14 days postoperatively. Secondary endpoints were length of hospital stay and duration of requirement for dressings.

Results.—Forty patients were included in the study analysis and completed self-reported pain and incapacity scores. Twenty received the fibrin sealant plus self-adhesive fabric dressing and 20 received the fabric dressing only (controls). Patients using the fibrin sealant plus the dressing reported significantly less pain (mean score, 0.42 versus 1.60, $p < 0.001$) and significantly less incapacity (mean score, 0.48 versus 1.71, $p < 0.001$). Patients allocated to the fibrin sealant group recorded shorter lengths of stay and faster time to discontinuation of dressing, though statistical significance was not achieved.

Conclusion.—Patients whose split skin graft donor sites were dressed with fibrin sealant plus self-adhesive fabric dressing experienced significantly less pain and incapacity than patients with self-adhesive fabric dressings alone, allowing a more rapid return to normal activity.

▶ Virtually all surgeons who perform skin grafts are well aware of the downside: creation of a secondary wound and the pain and incapacity associated with the donor site. Plastic surgeons and others have searched long and hard for the Holy Grail: artificial skin that might obviate the need for an autograft, or, failing that, the ability to take a skin graft with minimal morbidity at the donor site. This study does seem to address, at least in part, some of the challenges inherent in donor site morbidity, namely bleeding at the site, postoperative pain, and postoperative incapacity. The study single blinded, so that the patients were not aware if they did or did not receive the fibrin sealant. The outcomes, pain levels, and incapacities reported by the patients were found to be significantly better in the fibrin sealant group. Secondary outcomes were noted by the physicians and included length of hospital stay and discontinuation of dressings, and although the outcomes favored the fibrin group, the data did not reach statistical significance. The cost for the sealant is relatively low, and as long as patients are not allergic to the bovine substrate and the pooled human serum used to manufacture it is infection free, it should pose minimal risk. It would be interesting to repeat this study using more patients more rigorously matched for age and comorbidities (done to some extent in the reported study) and to double blind the study so as to allow a better analysis of secondary outcome data. This could easily be done by using a spray of saline randomized with a spray containing the active fibrin sealant.

S. H. Miller, MD

Flaps

Enhancement of Venous Drainage with Vein Stripper for Reversed Pedicled Neurocutaneous Flaps

Sonmez E, Silistireli ÖK, Karaaslan Ö, et al (Ataturk Res and Training Hosp, Izmir, Turkey; et al)

J Reconstr Microsurg 29:249-254, 2013

The flaps based on the vascular axis of superficial sensitive cutaneous nerves had gained increased popularity in reconstructive surgery because of such major advantages as preservation of major extremity arteries and avoidance of microsurgical procedures. However, postoperative venous congestion resulting in partial or total necrosis is still a common problem for these flaps. The aim of the current study is to introduce a new method for reducing the postoperative venous congestion of neural island flap with the results of reconstruction of the soft tissue defects of foot and ankle. This method was used to treat 19 patients with various chronic soft tissue defects of the foot and ankle between 2011 and 2012. We observed that the novel method presented in this report enables effective venous drainage, solving the postoperative venous congestion problem of these flaps.

▶ This is an interesting report apparently showing the benefits of destroying the valves in the lesser saphenous vein of a reverse sural island flap to minimize venous congestion. The report gives the results of 19 patients. Of those, 4 of 8 with diabetes, had minor wound dehiscence not further defined as to size, extent, and outcome. The technique involves a 2-stage procedure with a delay of 2 weeks. It is not clear to me that the beneficial effect was due entirely to the destruction of the valves of the lesser saphenous vein, or to the neovascularization secondary to the delay, or to some other factor(s). Obviously, further study will help clarify this issue.

S. H. Miller, MD

Microsurgery

Simulation of plastic surgery and microvascular procedures using perfused fresh human cadavers

Carey JN, Rommer E, Sheckter C, et al (Keck School of Medicine of the Univ of Southern California, Los Angeles, CA)
J Plast Reconstr Aesthet Surg 67:e42-e48, 2014

Introduction.—Surgical simulation models are often limited by their lack of fidelity, which hinders their essential purpose, making a better surgeon. Fresh cadaveric tissue is a superior model of simulation owing to its approximation of live tissue. One major unresolved difference between dead and live tissue is perfusion. Here, we propose a means of enhancing the fidelity of cadaveric simulation through the development of a perfused cadaveric model whereby simulation is further able to approach life-like surgery and teach one of the more technically demanding skills of plastic surgery: microsurgery.

Method.—Fresh tissue human cadavers were procured according to university protocol. Perfusion was performed via cannulation of large vessels, and arterial and venous pressure was maintained by centrifugal circulation. Skin perfusion was evaluated with incisions in the perfused regions and was evaluated using indocyanine green angiography. Surgical simulations were selected to broadly evaluate applicability to plastic surgical education.

Result.—Surgical simulation of 38 procedures ranging in complexity from skin excisions to microsurgical cases was performed with high priority given to the accurate simulation of clinical procedures. Flap dissections included perforator flaps, muscle flaps, and fasciocutaneous flaps. Effective perfusion was noted with ICG angiography and notable bleeding vessels. Microsurgical flap transfer was successfully performed.

Conclusion.—We report the establishment of a high fidelity surgical simulation using a perfused fresh tissue model in a realistic environment akin to the operating room. We anticipate utilization of this model prior to entering the operating room will enhance surgical ability and offer a valuable resource in plastic surgical education.

▶ Simulation is here to stay. It will become a routine part of medical student and resident education, a keystone in meeting the milestones, and probably part of board certification and recertification. Plastic surgery has been a relatively late adopter. This article is a nice initiation to simulation and to the specific needs of plastic surgery. The ability to confirm cutaneous circulation is important. The model also provides a lot of versatility for different procedures. This is an interesting concept to include in the overall simulation agenda.

D. J. Smith, Jr, MD

Collagen Conduit Versus Microsurgical Neurorrhaphy: 2-Year Follow-Up of a Prospective, Blinded Clinical and Electrophysiological Multicenter Randomized, Controlled Trial

Boeckstyns ME, Sørensen AI, Viñeta JF, et al (Univ of Copenhagen, Denmark; et al)

J Hand Surg Am 38:2405-2411, 2013

Purpose.—To compare repair of acute lacerations of mixed sensory-motor nerves in humans using a collagen tube versus conventional repair.

Methods.—In a prospective randomized trial, we repaired the ulnar or the median nerve with a collagen nerve conduit or with conventional microsurgical techniques. We enrolled 43 patients with 44 nerve lacerations. We performed electrophysiological tests and hand function using a standardized clinical evaluation instrument, the Rosen scoring system, after 12 and 24 months.

Results.—Operation time using the collagen conduit was significantly shorter than for conventional neurorrhaphy. There were no complications in terms of infection, extrusion of the conduit, or other local adverse reaction. Thirty-one patients with 32 nerve lesions, repaired with collagen conduits or direct suture, attended the 24-month follow-up. There was no difference between sensory function, discomfort, or total Rosen scores. Motor scores were significantly better for the direct suture group after 12 months, but after 24 months, there were no differences between the treatment groups. There was a general further recovery of both motor and sensory conduction parameters at 24 months compared with 12 months. There were no statistically significant differences in amplitudes, latencies, or conduction velocities between the groups.

Conclusions.—Use of a collagen conduit produced recovery of sensory and motor functions that were equivalent to direct suture 24 months after repair when the nerve gap inside the tube was 6 mm or less, and the collagen conduit proved to be safe for these nerve lacerations in the forearm.

▶ This study compares, in a prospective randomized trial, ulnar and median nerve lacerations repaired with a collagen nerve conduit or with conventional microsurgical techniques. Operating time was significantly shorter with the conduit. There were no conduit-associated complications. There was no difference between sensory function discomfort and total Rosen scores. At 24 months, the collagen conduit provided results comparable to those of direct repair, although direct repair achieved the results more rapidly. The gap was 6 months or less. Obviously, all of these injuries were amenable to direct repair, implying sharp clean injuries. I'm not sure I would extrapolate to other clinical situations based on these results.

D. J. Smith, Jr, MD

Facial allotransplantation: A 3-year follow-up report

Diaz-Siso JR, Parker M, Bueno EM, et al (Brigham and Women's Hosp, Boston, MA)

J Plast Reconstr Aesthet Surg 66:1458-1463, 2013

Introduction.—Long term follow-up of face transplant patients is fundamental to our understanding of risks and benefits of this procedure. Worldwide experience has shown that function improves gradually over time.

Methods.—In April of 2009, a multidisciplinary team at Brigham and Women's Hospital performed face transplantation on a male patient to address a severe facial defect caused by high-voltage burns. Physical and occupational therapy was performed for the first six post-operative months. Close monitoring of the patient's functional recovery, immunosuppression, and quality of life was performed at set time points.

Results.—Three years after face transplantation, the patient has recovered near-normal sensation. Along with satisfactory aesthetic results, his motor function continues to improve, aiding his speech, facial expressions, and social interaction. Furthermore, the patient reports continued improvements in quality of life. Infectious, metabolic, and immunologic complications have been successfully managed in a team approach. Immunosuppression doses have been effectively reduced, and steroid therapy was withdrawn before the end of the first postoperative year.

Conclusions.—The presented outcomes demonstrate the procedure's growing role in reconstructive surgery as teams continue to focus their efforts on further optimization of immunosuppression and surgical technique.

▶ These patients represent triumphs of technical surgical skill, but equally important is the presence and involvement of a dedicated team of health care specialists. Although individual case reports continue to be interesting to read and follow, much greater knowledge can and will be gained by the various centers pooling their data, especially long term. One such reason is that alluded to by these authors concerning the differences in experience when dealing with the need to coapt sensory nerves.[1] It would also be interesting to see if and when results become stable enough to reduce immunosuppression, to see when sensory and motor function stabilize, and to have some data on the overall costs involved in the treatment of these patients.

S. H. Miller, MD

Reference

1. Siemionow M, Gharb BB, Rampazzo A. Pathways of sensory recovery after face transplantation. *Plast Reconstr Surg*. 2011;127:1875-1889.

The role of the anterolateral thigh flap in complex defects of the scalp and cranium

Lin P-Y, Miguel R, Chew K-Y, et al (Kaohsiung Chang Gung Memorial Hosp and Chang Gung Univ College of Medicine, Taiwan; Kandang Kerbau Women's and Children's Hosp, Singapore)
Microsurgery 34:14-19, 2014

In this study, we introduced scalp reconstruction using free anterolateral thigh (ALT) flaps and evaluated postoperative outcomes in nine patients between March 2000 and April 2012. Five patients had problems of exposed prosthesis, three required reconstruction after resection of scalp tumor and one patient presented with third degree flame burns of the scalp. All flaps survived without re-exploration, except three flaps with tip necrosis requiring secondary procedures of debridement and small Z-plasty reconstructions. The superficial temporal artery and its concomitant vein were used as recipient vessels, apart from two cases where previous surgery and flame burns excluded these choices, for which facial arteries and veins were used instead. Primary closure of the donor-site was possible in six cases; with skin grafting performed for the other three patients. All donor sites healed without complications. The ALT flap offers the advantage of customizable size, option of fascia lata as vascularized dural replacement, and minimal flap atrophy typical of muscle flaps. Indications include very large defects, defects with exposed prosthesis, or defects with bone or dural loss. Our experience lends credible support to the use of customized free ALT flaps to achieve functional and cosmetically superior result for the reconstruction of large scalp defects, especially with bone exposure (Fig 5).

▶ One of the more appealing rationales for the use of the anterolateral thigh flap for scalp and cranial reconstruction is the availability of the fascia lata for reconstruction of the dura, should that be necessary. The ease of dissection is a plus as is the opportunity to close the donor site primarily if it is not larger than about 15% of the circumference of the thigh; however, in one-third of the

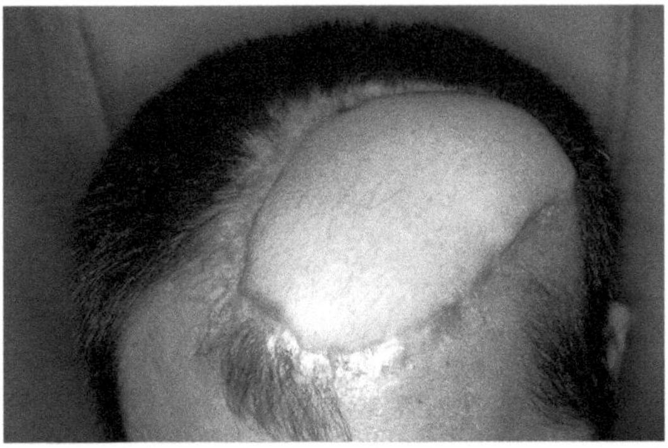

FIGURE 5.—The wound has healed without any major complication at 1-year follow-up. [Color figure can be viewed in the online issue, which is available at wileyonlinelibrary.com.] (Reprinted from Lin P-Y, Miguel R, Chew K-Y, et al. The role of the anterolateral thigh flap in complex defects of the scalp and cranium. *Microsurgery.* 2014;34:14-19, with permission from Microsurgery and Wiley-Liss, www.interscience.wiley.com.)

cases presented, it was not possible to close the donor defect without the use of skin grafts. In one-third of the cases presented, tip necrosis of the flap occurred, which required a secondary procedure. Finally, as with other flaps, this one tends to be a poor color match for the surrounding tissue, and the inevitable scar contracture resulting from filling a circular defect produces an unsightly bulge.

S. H. Miller, MD

Functional Restoration of Diaphragmatic Paralysis: An Evaluation of Phrenic Nerve Reconstruction

Kaufman MR, Elkwood AI, Colicchio AR, et al (Jersey Shore Univ Med Ctr, Neptune, NJ; The Inst for Advanced Reconstruction, Shrewsbury, NJ; et al)
Ann Thorac Surg 97:260-267, 2014

Background.—Unilateral diaphragmatic paralysis causes respiratory deficits and can occur after iatrogenic or traumatic phrenic nerve injury in the neck or chest. Patients are evaluated using spirometry and imaging studies; however, phrenic nerve conduction studies and electromyography are not widely available or considered; thus, the degree of dysfunction is often unknown. Treatment has been limited to diaphragmatic plication. Phrenic nerve operations to restore diaphragmatic function may broaden therapeutic options.

Methods.—An interventional study of 92 patients with symptomatic diaphragmatic paralysis assigned 68 (based on their clinical condition) to phrenic nerve surgical intervention (PS), 24 to nonsurgical (NS) care, and evaluated a third group of 68 patients (derived from literature review) treated with diaphragmatic plication (DP). Variables for assessment included spirometry, the Short-Form 36-Item survey, electrodiagnostics, and complications.

Results.—In the PS group, there was an average 13% improvement in forced expiratory volume in 1 second ($p < 0.0001$) and 14% improvement in forced vital capacity ($p < 0.0001$), and there was corresponding 17% ($p < 0.0001$) and 16% ($p < 0.0001$) improvement in the DP cohort. In the PS and DP groups, the average postoperative values were 71% for forced expiratory volume in 1 second and 73% for forced vital capacity. The PS group demonstrated an average 28% ($p < 0.01$) improvement in Short-Form 36-Item survey reporting. Electrodiagnostic testing in the PS group revealed a mean 69% ($p < 0.05$) improvement in conduction latency and a 37% ($p < 0.0001$) increase in motor amplitude. In the NS group, there was no significant change in Short-Form 36-Item survey or spirometry values.

Conclusions.—Phrenic nerve operations for functional restoration of the paralyzed diaphragm should be part of the standard treatment algorithm in the management of symptomatic patients with this condition. Assessment of neuromuscular dysfunction can aid in determining the most effective therapy.

▶ The authors conclude that phrenic nerve operations for functional restoration of the paralyzed diaphragm should be part of the standard treatment algorithm in the treatment of symptomatic patients with this condition. Assessment of neuromuscular dysfunction can aid in determining whether phrenic nerve repair or diaphragmatic plication is appropriate. The article is comprehensive and well worth reading for those doing microsurgery. What is interesting, and to some degree disappointing, is that no plastic surgeons were included. We have always survived and thrived by expanding our horizons. Maybe this and other nerve injuries provide another opportunity and challenge.

D. J. Smith, Jr, MD

Sequential free tissue transfers for simultaneous upper and lower limb salvage

Valerio IL, Sabino J, Bevevino A, et al (Walter Reed Natl Military Med Ctr, Bethesda, MD; et al)

Microsurgery 33:447-453, 2013

Background.—The Iraq and Afghanistan Wars have presented military reconstructive surgeons with a high volume of challenging extremity injuries. In recent years, a number of upper and lower extremity injuries requiring multiple tissue transfers for multiple limb salvages in the same casualty have been encountered. Our group will discuss the microsurgical challenges, algorithms, and success and complication rates for this cohort of war injured patients.

Methods.—All consecutive limb salvage cases requiring free flaps from 2003 to 2012 were reviewed. Cases involving simultaneous free tissue transfers were identified. Data collected included success rates and complications with comparisons made between the single and multiple free-flap limb salvage cohorts.

Results.—Seventy-four free flap limb salvage cases were performed over the 10-year period. Of these cases, four patients received two free flaps to separate upper and lower extremity injuries for limb salvage within a single operative setting. The complication rate was 63%, which was significantly higher than those cases in which a single microvascular anastomosis was performed (26%, $p = 0.046$). However, the higher complication rate did not increase the flap or limb salvage failure rates ($p = 0.892$ and 0.626).

Conclusions.—The last decade of war trauma has provided a high volume of extremity injuries requiring limb salvage procedures including casualties who underwent single and multiple free flap coverage procedures. Although multiple flap limb salvage procedures have a higher complication rate, they can be performed within the same patient without concern for increased failure rate in carefully selected and appropriately managed patients.

▶ War is awful, and there are few benefits ever. The injuries incurred are horrendous, resulting either in death or significant devastation. The force associated with the explosions from improvised explosive devices has created injuries never before seen. This article discusses lessons learned with extremity injuries requiring sequential free tissue transfers for simultaneous upper and lower limb salvage. They discuss the microsurgical challenges, algorithms, and success and complication rates for this cohort of war-injured patients. It is well worth learning from this unusual experience.

D. J. Smith Jr, MD

Outcome Measures of Microsurgical Toe Transfers for Reconstruction of Congenital and Traumatic Hand Anomalies

Kaplan JD, Jones NF (Shriners Hosp for Children, Los Angeles, CA)

J Pediatr Orthop 34:362-368, 2014

Background.—Outcomes data for children undergoing surgical reconstruction of their congenital hand anomalies has been used infrequently or not at all. Some surgeons even contend that children with total absence of digits or hands function perfectly well. Therefore, the purpose of this study was to evaluate and compare the functional outcomes of children who have undergone microsurgical toe-to-hand transfers for reconstruction of congenital and traumatic hand anomalies with the normal pediatric population.

Methods.—A total of 10 adolescents and 15 parents of pediatric and adolescent patients who underwent microsurgical toe-to-hand transfers were assessed using the Pediatric Outcomes Data Collection Instrument (PODCI) survey. Surveys were distributed during routine clinic visits or by mail. Indication and diagnosis were analyzed in relation to the functional outcomes obtained from the survey. Scores of the toe transfer patients group were compared with the scores of the normal pediatric population as well as the effect of patient and parent reporting.

Results.—Of the 3 survey groups and 6 functional dimensions, there was no statistically significant difference in function between the toe transfer children and the normal pediatric population in 13 of the 18 groups (72%). Adolescent toe transfer patients reported decreased upper extremity function and transfer/basic mobility and parents of adolescents reported decreased upper extremity function, sports/physical function, and global function. Parents significantly underestimated their adolescent children's function in terms of sports/physical function and happiness. Scores did not significantly differ between the congenital or traumatic indications for toe-to-hand transfers.

Conclusions.—Children with congenital or traumatic missing or hypoplastic digits who undergo reconstruction by microsurgical toe-to-hand transfer can achieve remarkable gains in function, sensation and ability to perform daily activities. This study confirms that a significant percentage of children undergoing reconstruction by microsurgical toe-to-hand transfers have similar functional outcomes assessments when compared withthe normal pediatric population.

Level of Evidence.—Level III—Therapeutic study.

▶ The purpose of this study was to evaluate and compare the functional outcomes of children who have undergone microsurgical toe-to-hand transfers for reconstruction of congenital and traumatic hand anomalies with those of the normal population. The study confirms that a significant percentage of children undergoing reconstruction by microsurgical toe-to-hand transfers have similar functional outcomes assessments when compared with the normal pediatric population. The authors used the Pediatric Outcomes Data Collection Instrument (PODCI). Although the numbers are small, the rigor of the analysis is excellent. This is a complete review with excellent outcomes parameters in function, sensation, and ability to perform activities of daily living.

D. J. Smith, Jr, MD

Analysis of multiple risk factors affecting the result of free flap transfer for necrotising soft tissue defects of the lower extremities in patients with type 2 diabetes mellitus

Kim BK, Lee YK, Park KY, et al (Seoul Natl Univ Bundang Hosp, Seongnam, Gyeonggi, Republic of Korea)

J Plast Reconstr Aesthet Surg 67:624-628, 2014

Background.—The limb-threatening large soft tissue defects that occur on the feet of type 2 diabetic patients have complex causes and are less likely to be corrected by free flap reconstruction compared to those in non-diabetic patients. We retrospectively analysed factors affecting the success of free flap transfer for necrotising soft tissue defects of the lower extremities in patients with type 2 diabetes.

Methods.—This study included 33 diabetic patients whose feet were treated with free flap transfers. All patients had limb-threatening large soft tissue defects with tendon or bone exposure. The operative results were divided into three groups at 1 month post-operatively: the complete healing group, and the complication group, with either partial necrosis requiring additional simple procedures or flap failure with total necrosis. Nine preoperative factors were analysed: (1) ankle brachial index, (2) HbA1c, (3) BMI, (4) the smoking factor, (5) atherosclerotic calcifications (6) serum creatinine levels ($>1.28\ mg\ dL^{-1}$ vs. $<1.28\ mg\ dL^{-1}$), (7) GFR, (8) wound infection and (9) wound defect size.

Results.—Of the 33 patients, 15 showed complete healing and 18 showed complications of the free flap (eight partial necrosis and 10 flap failure). No atherosclerotic calcifications were found in the patients in the complete healing group, although they were found in 12 patients in the complication group, and this difference was significant ($p = 0.002$). Patients with serum creatinine levels $>1.28\ mg\ dL^{-1}$ had significantly higher free flap transfer complication rates than those with serum creatinine levels $<1.28\ mg\ dL^{-1}$ ($p = 0.038$).

Conclusions.—This study analysed the risk factors of free flap reconstruction for limb-threatening large soft tissue defects on the feet of type 2 diabetic patients. Serum creatinine levels $>1.28\ mg\ dL^{-1}$ and atherosclerotic calcifications were confirmed as risk factors for flap survival.

▶ Type 2 diabetic patients with major soft tissue defects of the lower extremity are in great danger of losing the affected limb. Obviously with the ability to cover these defects with healthy donor tissues from elsewhere has encouraged many to try to prevent amputation and salvage these limbs. However, logic dictates that adequate vascular inflow to the effected area is essential if the flap is to survive and accomplish its intended purpose. The authors clearly show that atherosclerotic lesions pose a high risk of failure as does renal disease. One might ask whether the group of patients who underwent revascularization procedures before free-flap transfer actually had a stable vascular inflow for a period of time before performing the free flap. Another issue is whether the patients with elevated creatinine and low glomerular filtration rate were treated medically to try to reverse some of the effects of their renal disease. Larger series of patients should be studied to provide important data that will allow us to select, with a high degree of assurance, those who will benefit from these heroic efforts as opposed to those who will not.

S. H. Miller, MD

8 Miscellaneous

A Multicenter Randomized Controlled Trial Comparing Absorbable Barbed Sutures Versus Conventional Absorbable Sutures for Dermal Closure in Open Surgical Procedures

Rubin JP, Hunstad JP, Polynice A, et al (Univ of Pittsburgh Med Ctr, PA; Univ of North Carolina, Chapel Hill; Albany Med Ctr, NY; et al)

Aesthet Surg J 34:272-283, 2014

Background.—Barbed sutures were developed to reduce operative time and improve security of wound closure.

Objective.—The authors compare absorbable barbed sutures (V-Loc, Covidien, Mansfield, Massachusetts) with conventional (smooth) absorbable sutures for soft tissue approximation.

Method.—A prospective multicenter randomized study comparing barbed sutures with smooth sutures was undertaken between August 13, 2009, and January 31, 2010, in 241 patients undergoing abdominoplasty, mastopexy, and reduction mammaplasty. Each patient received barbed sutures on 1 side of the body, with deep dermal sutures eliminated or reduced. Smooth sutures with deep dermal and subcuticular closure were used on the other side as a control. The primary endpoint was dermal closure time. Safety was assessed through adverse event reporting through a 12-week follow-up.

Results.—A total of 229 patients were ultimately treated (115 with slow-absorbing polymer and 114 with rapid-absorbing polymer). Mean dermal closure time was significantly quicker with the barbed suture compared with the smooth suture (12.0 vs 19.2 minutes; $P < .001$), primarily due to the need for fewer deep dermal sutures. The rapid-absorbing barbed suture showed a complication profile equivalent to the smooth suture, while the slow-absorbing barbed suture had a higher incidence of minor suture extrusion.

Conclusions.—Barbed sutures enabled faster dermal closure quicker than smooth sutures, with a comparable complication profile.

Level of Evidence.—1.

▶ Barbed sutures are ideal for plastic surgery procedures that have long incisions or some skin closure tension. This study confirms that an average of 5 minutes is saved for common long-incision closures. Each surgeon must decide if the additional time savings is worth the increased suture cost.

K. A. Gutowski, MD

The Beneficial Effects of Postrhinoplasty Taping: Fact or Fiction?

Belek KA, Gruber RP (Alta Bates Summit Med Ctr, Oakland, CA; Stanford Univ, CA)

Aesthet Surg J 34:56-60, 2014

Background.—Initial patient perceptions of rhinoplasty results are complicated by early postoperative edema, ecchymosis, and distortion. Anecdotal evidence suggests that taping the nose immediately upon splint removal aids with the patient's psychological adjustment to his or her new appearance.

Objectives.—The authors attempt to assess the overall impact of taping after splint removal on patient well-being while providing statistical validation regarding the utility of this intervention.

Methods.—The authors evaluated the reaction of 24 postoperative rhinoplasty patients on the day of splint removal by photographing them and noting their verbal responses. Those patients who were obviously happy received no taping and were dismissed from the study. The remainder of the patients received flesh-colored tape (3M, St Paul, Minnesota) and their subsequent reactions were noted and photographed.

Results.—Of 24 consecutive patients, 16 received tape. Fifteen of those taped initially displayed a flat affect (group A), while 1 was clearly unhappy (group B). The remaining 8 patients were obviously happy (group C) and were excluded from taping. Thirteen (86%) of those in group A displayed immediate subjective improvement after taping ($\chi^2 = 12.8$; $P < .001$). The lone patient in group B continued to be unhappy and required ongoing reassurance.

Conclusions.—Application of tape immediately upon splint removal after rhinoplasty improves initial patient perceptions. Taping can provide a simple and risk-free intervention for patients who do not express immediate satisfaction.

▶ Although it may sound silly, an extra week of covering the nose with tape instead of a splint may help a patient adjust better to their rhinoplasty results. The authors call this a psychological bridge that provides a limited view of the nose and allows for a few more days of coverage while swelling and bruising resolve.

K. A. Gutowski, MD

From the Operating Room to the Courtroom: A Comprehensive Characterization of Litigation Related to Facial Plastic Surgery Procedures

Svider PF, Keeley BR, Zumba O, et al (Univ of Medicine and Dentistry of New Jersey, Newark; Mount Sinai School of Medicine, NY; et al)

Laryngoscope 123:1849-1853, 2013

Objectives/Hypothesis.—Malpractice litigation has increased in recent decades, contributing to higher health-care costs. Characterization of complications leading to litigation is of special interest to practitioners of facial plastic surgery procedures because of the higher proportion of elective cases relative to other subspecialties. In this analysis, we comprehensively examine malpractice litigation in facial plastic surgery procedures and characterize factors important in determining legal responsibility, as this information may be of great interest and use to practitioners in several specialties.

Study Design.—Retrospective analysis.

Methods.—The Westlaw legal database was examined for court records pertaining to facial plastic surgery procedures. The term "medical malpractice" was searched in combination with numerous procedures obtained from the American Academy of Facial Plastic and Reconstructive Surgery website.

Results.—Of the 88 cases included, 62.5% were decided in the physician's favor, 9.1% were resolved with an out-of-court settlement, and 28.4% ended in a jury awarding damages for malpractice. The mean settlement was $77,437 and mean jury award was $352,341. The most litigated procedures were blepharoplasties and rhinoplasties. Alleged lack of informed consent was noted in 38.6% of cases; other common complaints were excessive scarring/disfigurement, functional considerations, and postoperative pain.

Conclusions.—This analysis characterized factors in determining legal responsibility in facial plastic surgery cases. Several factors were identified as potential targets for minimizing liability. Informed consent was the most reported entity in these malpractice suits. This finding emphasizes the importance of open communication between physicians and their patients regarding expectations as well as documentation of specific risks, benefits, and alternatives.

▶ As with the medical-legal analysis of body contouring, patient–physician communication and the informed consent process are cited as key issues in legal action after facial plastic surgery. However, in these cases, functional problems related to blepharoplasty and rhinoplasty were also common.

K. A. Gutowski, MD

Beyond the Operating Room: A Look at Legal Liability in Body Contouring Procedures

Paik AM, Mady LJ, Sood A, et al (Rutgers Univ, Newark, NJ)

Aesthet Surg J 34:106-113, 2014

Background.—Malpractice claims affect the cost and quality of health care.

Objective.—In this study, the authors examine legal litigation following body contouring surgery and identify factors influencing malpractice litigation outcomes.

Methods.—The Westlaw legal database was searched for jury verdict and settlement reports related to body contouring procedures and medical malpractice. Cases included for analysis were examined for year of report, geographic location, patient demographics, procedure performed, alleged injury, causes of action, verdict, and indemnity payments.

Results.—Of 113 cases, the most common injuries sustained were disfigurement (33.6%) and the necessitation of a revision procedure (33.6%). The most common cause of action cited was negligence (84.1%). Median plaintiff ages differed significantly ($P = .003$) between cases favoring the defendant (44.5 years) and those favoring the plaintiff (36 years). Of the alleged injuries, those cases citing an iatrogenic injury were 2.5 times more likely to result in either damages awarded or settlement (relative risk [RR], 2.5; 95% confidence interval [CI], 1.66-3.80). Cases that cited disfigurement were 87% more likely to result in damages awarded to the plaintiff (RR, 1.87; 95% CI, 1.08-3.26).

Conclusions.—Based on this study of body contouring litigation, younger plaintiff age and iatrogenic injury strongly favored plaintiffs in either awarded damages or a settlement. Disfigurement favored plaintiffs only in awarded damages. Our study emphasizes the need for adequate communication with the patient explaining realistic aesthetic results and risks of the procedure. In addition, iatrogenic organ injury must be handled expeditiously. Incorporating these recommendations into clinical practice may promote an improved physician-patient relationship while reducing litigatious health care costs.

▶ This medical-legal case review underscores the importance of surgeon—patient communication, proper informed consent process (consisting of documented patient education and understanding of risks and outcomes), and patient selection with assessment for realistic expectations. Although not all adverse outcomes and legal actions can be prevented, attention to these points may lessen the chance of a legal claim.

K. A. Gutowski, MD

Article Index

Chapter 1: Congenital

Chapter 2: Neoplastic, Inflammatory and Degenerative Conditions

Chapter 3: Trauma

Chapter 4: Hand and Upper Extremity

Chapter 5: Aesthetic

Chapter 6: Breast

Chapter 7: Grafts, Flaps, and Microsurgery

Chapter 8: Miscellaneous

Author Index

FSC
www.fsc.org
MIX
Papier | Fördert gute Waldnutzung
FSC® C083411

Kolibri 360 GmbH
Ferdinand-Jühlke-Straße 7
99095 Erfurt, Deutschland
produktsicherheit@kolibri360.de